D1569480

To Be a Therapist:
The Teaching and Learning

+++

To Be a Therapist:

The Teaching and Learning

++

Jerry M. Lewis, M.D.

Timberlawn Psychiatric Hospital
Timberlawn Psychiatric Research Foundation
Dallas, Texas

BRUNNER/MAZEL, *Publishers* • New York

Library of Congress Cataloging in Publication Data

Lewis, Jerry M.   1924-
  To be a therapist.

  Includes bibliographical references and index.
  1. Psychotherapy—Study and teaching.   I.   Title.
RC480.5.L49   616.8'914'07   77-15035
ISBN 0-87630-153-7

MANUFACTURED IN THE UNITED STATES OF AMERICA

To Pat

With and For Love

The beginning, as the proverb says, is half the whole, so that a bad start does as much harm as all the later mistakes put together.

ARISTOTLE

CONTENTS

INTRODUCTION

+++

All psychotherapists are aware of the concept of overdetermination, the theory that a single act has a variety of determinants that often occupy different levels of awareness. Describing in written form the evolution and current status of an approach to teaching psychotherapeutic skills has led me to consider my personal investment in the teaching, as well as the source of that motivation. Although the final chapter of this book addresses the contextual factors that both permitted and nourished the seminar, unmistakably it has taken personal investment, drive, and need on my part to sustain it. I wish to share this personal motivation with the reader because I suspect that I am not alone in my response to the situation that pressed me.

First, I believe that, as a group, we, the teachers of psychotherapy, do an inadequate job of starting trainees on the road to competence. We throw them in the deep water of treating troubled patients at a tender age and help them, only in retrospect, to learn from their errors. We know so much more than what we teach beginners that it is tempting to think that we are caught up in a not-too-subtle initiation process: We survived the rites, and the next generation will be somehow as strong or stronger if they face the same anxieties and stresses. In the years since our own beginnings as therapists, however, we have learned much through our collective experiences and a variety of research efforts. This information can be translated into teaching exercises that provide the beginner with, at the minimum, some understanding of both what therapists do specifically and the rationale behind their methods. We can do this in a way that incorporates the best of science and current knowledge. In Beavers' (1) words, we need be neither doctrinaire nor evangelical about one particular approach, but we do owe our students an open presentation of the theory and techniques of all major contributors. I believe that the introduction to psychotherapeutic techniques is of particular importance at the very beginning of the students' training. Logically, it should occupy as significant an early position as individual supervision and personal psychotherapy or psychoanalysis may come to occupy throughout the trainees' education.

At a different level, however, I am aware that my investment in this type of teaching reflects also my frequent dissatisfaction with the results of my own psychotherapeutic activity. After a few years of psychotherapeutic practice, I became increasingly incredulous that a process of such strength could result in sweeping life changes for some and no change for others. (At that point in my evolution as a therapist, I was unable to think in terms of the *worsening* of some patients' lives as the result of psychotherapy.) How could something potentially so helpful often fail? My response, similar I would guess to that of other therapists, was to obtain supervision, read widely, attend seminars, and to think and ponder that which my teachers and supervisors had taught me. Ultimately, I decided that I had to learn more—that, most of all, it was necessary to understand the process of psychotherapeutic failure and to recognize its form early enough to avoid its conclusion. There was no psychoanalytic institute in my community; if there had been, I strongly suspect that it would have received my application, for that training offered the promise of greater learning. At this time, I began taping some of my psychotherapy interviews and requested supervisees to do the same. In restrospect, the seminar started with the purchase of a tape recorder, but it was pushed by my need to know more about effective psychotherapy. In effect, part of my motivation to teach was to learn.

In discussing this issue with colleagues who are close friends, I find others share this concern about the failures of a process that has such potential for good. My position on the staff of a private hospital with a residency training program, however, provided the setting in which my concern could be translated into a seminar.

During the years in which the seminar has evolved, there has been considerable change in its emphasis. Most broadly, the initial years focused almost exclusively on affect and the development of empathic skills. During more recent years, the central emphasis has been on the balance of intimacy and detachment and the fluctuation between these positions during the course of each psychotherapy interview. Currently, the seminar commences with a focus on empathy, but moves on to consider the skills involved in the therapist's ability to understand and intervene with the patient.

Throughout the seminar, however, there has been an enduring commitment to experiential learning. In "doing" what therapists do, the students inevitably disclose themselves and make mistakes. This arouses considerable affect. This arousal, however, is considered an important component of the learning that occurs, for sustained learning is most apt to occur in the educational setting (as in the therapeutic setting) when there is considerable affect involved.

The following description of the seminar does not purport to review meticulously the vast literature on psychotherapy, nor even the much smaller literature on the training of psychotherapists. The references to other teachers and writers are selective; these are the individuals and groups with whom I have corresponded or whose writings I have read. As a result, I am mindful that I have neglected other significant contributions.

The description of the seminar is offered, not as any type of ultimate solution or even preferred form of teaching psychotherapeutic skills, but rather as one offering to what should be the continuous process by which we, the teachers of psychotherapy, share our efforts and refine our craft. In addition, I am hopeful that the learning that has occurred for me in the teaching will be of assistance to other experienced psychotherapists in their struggle to achieve greater competence.

REFERENCE

1. BEAVERS, W. R., *Psychotherapy and Growth: A Family Systems Perspective.* New York: Brunner/Mazel, 1977.

ACKNOWLEDGMENTS

Books are written by individuals in certain contexts, and this one is no exception. My colleagues at the Timberlawn Psychiatric Hospital have provided me with both the freedom and the encouragement to experiment with teaching psychotherapeutic skills. In particular, the clinical leadership provided by James K. Peden, M.D., Howard M. Burkett, M.D., Doyle I. Carson, M.D., Byron L. Howard, M.D., Keith H. Johansen, M.D., Joe W. King, M.D., Charles G. Markward, M.D., and Larry E. Tripp, M.D., has provided me with time to experiment.

My research colleagues in the study of healthy families at the Timberlawn Psychiatric Research Foundation have provided another type of input. John T. Gossett, Ph.D., has been a source of encouragement, a friend and clinical colleague, and an enthusiastic and astute collaborator. W. Robert Beavers, M.D., has provided an unusual source of intellectual stimulation and excitement. Virginia Austin Phillips has encouraged, challenged and, more often than not, pushed me to sharpen and focus. In addition, she has provided major editorial and administrative support. Nannette Bruchey has endured all the changes, typed each draft, and by her competence has allowed me to range from teacher to therapist to researcher.

The resident psychiatrists, graduate students, and research assistants who have participated in the seminar are too numerous to mention. They have been, however, the heart of the seminar. Their willingness to risk self-esteem in an open educational process has provided the feedback that led to sequential modifications in the seminar.

In an even more intimate context, my children, Jerry M. Lewis III, M.D., Cynthia J. Lewis, Nancy J. Lewis, and Thomas P. Lewis have provided needed encouragement. Pat, my wife, to whom the book is dedicated, has sustained me through the preoccupation and detachment that go with writing, at the same time offering understanding, patience and warm support.

CHAPTER 1

Evolution of the Seminar

+‡+

There is wide agreement that becoming a psychotherapist is a long and difficult undertaking. The beginners are first-year residents in psychiatry and graduate students in psychology and social work. Their search to achieve and improve psychotherapeutic competence may last a professional lifetime. There are three sources of learning available during the initial stages of training: individual supervision, personal psychotherapy or psychoanalysis, and instruction in psychotherapeutic technique. If the beginner learns well from each of these experiences, he or she is better able to learn from patients who will continue this instruction in the most illuminating way of all.

This book describes a seminar in psychotherapeutic skills that the author has developed over a ten-year period. This first-year course in a psychiatric residency program has been enriched by the participation of students in other health disciplines.* **The plan of study has included selected readings and psychotherapy films of well-known therapists, but its focus has been primarily experiential—that is, doing what therapists do.**

As the seminar continues to evolve each year, the scope and emphases change. I like to think of the process of the seminar over time as one of distillation in which some of current knowledge of techniques can be clarified and made available. I believe that effective psychotherapy is a remarkable process of great power. Although our understanding of the factors responsible for the effectiveness of psychotherapy is as yet fragmentary, I also believe, along with Chessick (1, 2), that traditional methods of psychotherapeutic training do not present all that we know—there is a curious gap between knowledge and training methods. This seminar is an attempt to reduce that gap.

Many psychotherapeutic training programs place heavy, or even sole, emphasis on individual supervision as the learning experience. Some encourage or insist that beginning therapists undergo personal therapy. Few, however, make any major commitment of curriculum time to learning specific psychotherapeutic techniques. As a consequence, a more-or-less typical situation for the beginning therapist involves his or her seeing a patient "in therapy," taking notes, or writing a summary, and then presenting these data to a supervisor. This post hoc process (do it and then talk about it) is remarkable when contrasted with learning skills in other areas. Learning to be a psychotherapist is at least as complicated, for example, as learning to fly a jet plane. Few would recommend that a beginning pilot take off and fly a jet plane, only later to discuss with an instructor how and why the plane behaved the way it did. It seems equally useful to ask that beginning therapists have considerable preliminary instruction in the how and why of psychotherapy before they begin their actual psychotherapeutic work. The failure of many training programs to teach psychotherapeutic techniques systematically probably reflects a number of factors. The first may

---

* Students have been from the disciplines of psychology, social work, psychiatric nursing, and pastoral counseling.

be that few teachers were themselves recipients of such instruction. Most went into their initial hours of doing therapy with considerable anxiety and very little in the way of knowledge of specific techniques. Graduates of psychoanalytic institutes, of course, are an exception, but many teachers of psychotherapists feel that teaching psychoanalytic techniques is the business of psychoanalytic institutes exclusively, rather than of psychotherapy training programs. Another reason most training programs disregard the area of technique may be the lack of clarity about *what* to teach or *how* to teach specific skills. The situation has not improved since Matarazzo, Wiens, and Saslow (3) reviewed the literature ten years ago and wrote. "... there is essentially no published research regarding the teaching of psychotherapy, ... how learning of effective psychotherapy takes place and how to teach psychotherapy efficiently."

Another apparent resistance to teaching psychotherapeutic techniques is the tendency of some teachers to depreciate any concern with "how to do it" as a reflection of an inadequate appreciation of the richness and depth of human behavior. This criticism is superficial, overlooking the interdependence between theory and technique. Even Freud is said to have been influenced often by matters of technique, which then led to further refinements in theory (4). Finally, some training programs are led by individuals with a primary interest in other systems with which the discipline concerns itself (for example, delivery of services to large groups of people, as in community mental health centers), and their curricula will reflect these interests or commitments. Each training program certainly has the right to establish its own hierarchy of core skills within its field. Yet many mental health professionals will spend a considerable part of their professional lives as psychotherapists, and the achievement of an adequate level of psychotherapeutic competence upon completion of training should be a broadly agreed upon goal for all training programs.

The seminar to be described grew out of my personal dissatisfaction with conventional supervisory procedures, and I subsequently requested that those residents, graduate students, and practicing professionals whom I was supervising make audiotape recordings of their interviews. I also recorded some of my own interviews and became increasingly interested in psychotherapy that appeared to be stalemated. As one might expect, many different factors were involved in the bogged-down psychotherapy: Transference and countertransference issues, inadequate assessment of the patient's psychopathology, and inattention of the therapist in dealing with anxieties that intersected with his own are but a few examples. A surprisingly common finding, however, in stalemated psychotherapy was the therapist's failure to attend the patient's affect. In many such interviews, patients communicated intense feelings that were disregarded by the therapist who focused almost exclusively on the *content* of their fantasies, thoughts, or dreams. Interviews of this sort developed a sterile, intellectual, problem-solving quality. Often, the therapist sounded remote and appeared to be interested only in the "facts."

This observation of the interviews of numerous supervisees (as well as my own) led to an interest in how to increase the therapist's attention to feelings. A search of the writings about affect in psychotherapy included a broad literature on the value of empathy. Although definitions of therapist's empathy differed from one school of psychiatry to another, many writers described empathy as a central or indispensable therapist characteristic. It therefore appeared surprising that there was little about *how* to learn to be empathic. However, the work of Rogers, Truax, and Carkhuff (5, 6, 7) offered a structure with which to begin teaching specific skills.

It seemed important to offer this course early in the students' training and, if possible, before they began their initial psychotherapeutic work with patients. It was my hope that this would provide the students with a sense of the importance of feelings in psychotherapy and would reduce the possibility that students and their patients would be caught up in stalemated or nonproductive psychotherapy.

During the first course, I met with first-year residents and graduate students one hour a week, and we experimented with some exercises designed to increase a therapist's sensitivity to affective messages. The students responded to some typical, audiotaped patient statements, and the level of empathy in their responses was scored by the use of rating scales devised by Carkhuff (7). Gradually, other specific variables important in a therapist were added to the course, such as warmth, genuineness, specificity, and self-disclosure. At a later point in the evolution of the seminar, as the value of having an opportunity to use and assess specific techniques became clear, techniques from psychoanalytic psychotherapy were added. These included following trains of associations, the recognition of mechanisms of defense, and dealing with resistances. Recently, it has proved useful to emphasize the nonverbal factors in psychotherapy and the system aspects of the interview. This two-person interaction in which the therapist and the patient participate is seen to have observable and definable system characteristics. The research study of communication patterns of healthy families (8) suggested the nature of the system variables one should attend, and a colleague, W. Robert Beavers (9) has articulated that which healthy families in particular may teach individual therapists about their craft.

The focus of the seminar has broadened to include instruction in a wide range of variables thought to be related to effective psychotherapy. The sources included objective-descriptive psychiatry, existential psychiatry, interpersonal psychiatry, psychoanalytic theory and practice, and the study of effective or competent human systems. Throughout the seminar, the major emphasis has been experiential. The students see demonstrations, rehearse, discuss, practice, assess others, and are themselves assessed. The initial material they deal with involves audiotaped patient statements which they respond to at first in writing and, at a later stage, in spoken and recorded form. Next, videotape patient statements are used as an introduction to the increasing complexity of communication. Later, each of the students interviews the same actor "patient," and the videotapes of each interview are studied by the group with particular emphasis on the way an interviewer influences the direction of the interview. The students practice the use of techniques through role playing, and these interviews are observed and criticized by the group. Visual stimuli incorporating human needs, drives, and developmental phases are presented, and each student is asked to write a fantasy in response to the material. The fantasies are shared and the ways in which each individual may differ from his or her colleagues are noted. This exercise is an attempt to sensitize the students to the interactional base of psychotherapy and the need to be aware of their idiosyncratic responses and their potential impact upon the therapeutic interaction. Each is encouraged, for example, not to invite certain behavior and then label it as characteristic of the patient.

After approximately six months of preliminary experiential exercises, the students have been introduced to a dozen or so factors or processes that are central to various types of psychotherapy, and the focus of the course changes to patient interviews. Each student is involved in a number of interviews, which the group watches from behind a one-way mirror. Each student observer is asked to note one or two aspects of the interview. For example, one may rate the level of therapeutic empathy. Another is asked to report on the nonverbal behavior of both patient and therapist. Another is asked to observe the patient's defense mechanisms and report the observations that led to the identification of certain behavior as defensive. Others have comparable tasks. The students are encouraged to be open and candid. Under most circumstances they are, and the training is experienced as an honest and often painful experience, but rarely as one in which the individual feels attacked personally.

At this point in the student's training, he or she becomes therapist for three patients and is assigned to a supervisor for each patient. The students record all psychotherapy sessions on audiotapes, and generally take those tape recordings and a written summary of each interview to the supervisory session. The data, therefore, of the supervisory session are both the resident's summary and the actual verbatim tape recordings.

The major thrust of the course is the introduction of the students to many of the constructs involved in the process of therapy in a way that emphasizes learning through doing prior to the assumption of the role of psychotherapist. If there is something novel about this approach to training, it is the time and energy devoted to this initial stage of training. At the present time, the seminar is a four-hour-per-week, 200-hour first-year course.*

It is assumed, and over time has been noted, that each student puts together the various techniques or skills in a different way. There is no attempt to present a single, narrowly defined model of a therapist. Rather, the message is: "Here are what seem to be important processes associated with being an effective therapist. Examine them, understand them, take them out of context and practice them, and then, over time, put them all together in your own way. At first the use of some of them will seem artificial, and it will take time for that to change, to feel that they are a part of you. As these processes come to feel like a part of you, you are becoming a therapist."

WHAT TO TEACH?

One of the difficulties in teaching psychotherapeutic techniques in some systematic way is the uncertainty about what to teach. The field of psychotherapy is one of conflicting claims, as there are many schools, and each school suggests that its approach is the only way. The beginning therapist may be confused by these rivalries, and it is easy to fall captive to one teacher's particular ideology. This confusion may grow if the teacher makes no effort either to contrast the techniques of each school or to search for commonalities among them.

Bromberg (10) describes two groups of writers who are interested in psychotherapeutic technique. The first group, the "lumpers," searches for that which is common to all psychotherapies. The second group, the "splitters," emphasizes the differences between the schools. He cites Frank (11) as an outstanding example of a lumper who compares a wide variety of techniques known to result in basic attitudinal change. Psychotherapy is con-

---

* A more detailed outline of the seminar is presented in the appendix.

sidered along with processes as different as brainwashing, religious healing, and the placebo effect. Frank suggests that all of these processes share a group of four common variables: 1) A patient-therapist relationship in which the patient has confidence in the therapist's competence and feels that the therapist genuinely cares about his welfare. This feeling of acceptance and of being cared about is based upon the therapist's empathic understanding. 2) A setting that is sanctioned by cultural values and arouses the patient's expectation of help. 3) A rationale that includes an explanation of both illness and health. 4) A procedure or technique suitable to the theory.

These four features influence the patient to change in five interrelated ways: 1) They lead to increased emotional arousal. 2) They provide new opportunities for experiential and cognitive learning. 3) They increase the patient's hope of relief. 4) Provision for successful problem solving leads to an increased sense of competence and mastery. 5) The process itself aids in overcoming the previous demoralizing sense of alienation from others.

Frank states that the four features shared by all psychotherapies far outweigh their differences. Although that may be both true and important, the features are sufficiently broad as to be of modest value in training psychotherapists. They may best be thought of as important orienting generalities rather than specific learnable qualities for the beginning therapist.

Bromberg's "splitters" are of greater help in deciding what needs to be taught. This is because a careful differentiation of the techniques of each school leads to increased clarity about the use of techniques. Most splitters, however, present their descriptions in the fashion of protagonists, and both the student and teacher are apt to get caught up in a struggle that appears to involve a splitter's concern with demonstrating the superiority of his own school.

To this arena have come the outstanding contributions of Havens (12, 13, 14). In a series of books and articles, he has brought dispassionate clarity to this field. Havens describes four major psychotherapeutic approaches: the objective-descriptive, the psychoanalytic, the interpersonal, and the existential. He describes the techniques and clarifies the ideology and historical development of each school.

The objective-descriptive school is the oldest school and most clearly related to the traditional medical orientation of focusing on disease. The patient is seen as the bearer of a disease, and there is no major concern with the patient as a person. The therapist is concerned with the signs and the symptoms of the disease, and interviews are characterized by the therapist's focused questions as he or she attempts to arrive at a diagnostic level of understanding. Treatment is based upon this diagnostic level of understanding, and relies heavily upon encouraging, advising, and controlling the patient. The therapist is the authority, and he or she examines the patient in an "objective" way. Havens likens this model to a detective (doctor) looking for a criminal (disease).

The psychoanalytic approach represents a major step in the evolution of psychotherapy. There is a primary concern with the patient's inner mental life and, in particular, fantasies. The major techniques involve encouraging free associations, interpretations of resistances to those associations, and interpretation of transference. The therapist is less active than in the objective-descriptive school, and remains neutral. The psychoanalyst has a special interest in the influence of the past upon the present, and sees insight as the major vehicle of change. Rather than being preoccupied with disease as is the objective-descriptive therapist, he or she seeks to dissect the neurotic formations free from the personality and, in conjunction with the patient's mature ego, wear away their power.

Havens (13, p. 121) suggests that both existential psychotherapy and interpersonal psychiatry developed as a result of dissatisfaction with psychoanalysis as "too intellectual, too neutral, too passive, too concerned with fantasy at the expense of reality, too concerned with sexual elements at the expense of values and social relationships."

Existential psychiatry is concerned centrally with the *forms* rather than the content of inner experience. The technique requires the therapist to feel deeply with the patient without preconception or expectation. This is termed "being" and "staying," and it is important to note that this technique is an objective in itself rather than a method of obtaining data through associations. Indeed, the failure to collect data or to form conclusions about the patient is seen by others as the principal shortcoming of an existential therapist. There are, in effect, no objectives other than being and staying with the patient. Accordingly, what the patient says is taken at face value, and there is no search for any underlying meaning. Rather, the therapist attempts to translate the patient's current inner experience into words. At its core, the existential method is built upon a deep and pervasive empathy which permits the therapist to disclose his or her own feelings and thoughts when they are in the service of being with the patient. Havens indicates that this method gives the therapist the first systematic guide to self-disclosure. The existential method, then, focuses on feelings, reduces the distance between patient and therapist, requires maximum subjectivity rather than neutrality and objectivity, and suggests that countertransference issues are to be worked out within the relationship rather than silently in the therapist.

Interpersonal or social psychiatry focuses on the relationships of the patient and the social field in which the patient is a participant. The patient is seen as an individual with distorting assumptions (misunderstandings, projections, or parataxes) that drastically color relationships and communications with others. The therapist operates with a "fictive attitude," acting as if everything encountered clinically is fiction until proven fact. The therapist does not interpret the patient's distortions about the therapist; rather, without humiliating the patient, the therapist moves against them with counterprojective techniques. The role of the therapist is to act against these assumptions in the here-and-now of the relationship with the patient. The central questions for the therapist are, "What is the patient up to?" and "How can I respond in a way that makes the distortion about me untenable?" Fundamentally, interpersonal psychiatry is concerned with social reality—indeed, Havens (13) says, interpersonalists are as apt to blame everything on reality as psycho-analysts are to see everything as fantasy.

Each of the approaches espouses a particular focus, causal mechanisms, optimal type of relationship with the patient, ideals of health, and a group of techniques. The techniques of each school are based on selective data that confirm the school's basic propositions. Each evolved in response to many factors, not the least of which was the nature of the predominant psychopathology of a given historical period: Objective-descriptive psychiatry developed when organic states were a major focus of pyschiatry; psychoanalysis seems particularly related historically to the treatment of hysteria; existential psychiatry was responsive to the disturbances of severe psychopathology characterized by massive denial; and interpersonal psychiatry was evolved to meet the problems of treating major projective disturbances. There are numerous variants of each school, and each has practitioners currently functioning as competent therapists. Havens calls for a pluralism in psychiatry in which each therapist would be competent in the techniques of all schools and use whichever approach appears best suited to the individual patient. This is a goal to be reached for, but the current reality suggests that typically a therapist evolves a personal amalgam of techniques that suits his or her temperament, and that the psychoanalytic approach probably dominates this composite.

My own experience suggests that many therapists undergo a sequence similar to the evolution of the four major approaches Havens describes (a type of ontogeny recapitulating phylogeny). Psychiatrists, for example, start with the medical, disease-oriented model, examining the patient, noting the signs and symptoms of his disturbance, and making a definite diagnosis. A few psychiatrists continue to rely solely on this objective-descriptive model. Early in training, however, they are exposed to psychoanalytic theory and technique, and most incorporate a psychoanalytic model of psychotherapy. Eventually, some therapists move toward a more interpersonal or existential approach as their experience teaches them that the objective-descriptive and psychoanalytic approaches do not work well with all patients.

A few reject the approaches and techniques of earlier periods of professional development completely (often passionately), but many continue to add techniques which may be used selectively with patients.

A relatively new source of help in the training of psychotherapists is the study of optimal human systems. Our study of healthy families (8) focuses on families who accomplish the two cardinal purposes of families—the stabilization or continued growth of parental personalities and the production of healthy, autonomous children—with high levels of competence. Their relationship patterns, communication styles, and problem-solving techniques have particular relevance as a model for effective growth-oriented psychotherapy (9). This latter system quality is closely parallel to the process of psychotherapy: The therapist hopes to help the patient become healthy and autonomous. Several factors seem of particular importance. The first has to do with power or interpersonal influence. Healthy families share power; there is no dominant, all-powerful individual, but rather family members are collaborative, and each participates in the family's efforts to solve problems by negotiation. Dominant-submissive, conflicted, or chaotic patterns of interpersonal influence are characteristic of dysfunctional human systems which make human growth difficult. Healthy families suggest to the therapist that the therapist-patient relationship be collaborative in the sense that power is shared. In such a relationship, the therapist would not insist that his reality is the only valid one, but would understand that each person may see things differently. In the commitment to this subjective reality, the therapist both respects the patient's individual boundaries and offers a model of respect for such boundaries. The meaning of the patient's behavior is negotiated by both participants rather than proclaimed by the therapist. Listening and watching collaborative therapy interviews, one is impressed how often the therapist invites the patient to explore further a feeling, fantasy, or memory. It is obvious that the therapist really believes that greater understanding and behavioral change can be achieved if the patient is encouraged to probe deeper within himself or herself. The inevitable resistances are noted and clarified. The flow of such interviews, however, more clearly comes from the patient's feelings and associations. The occasions upon which the therapist must abandon collaboration and "take care of" the patient are rare. Severe toxic states or suicidal crises may be examples of situations that call for a protective or parental therapist position. Even in such situations, however, a therapist may involve the patient in the decision-making to some degree.

Luborsky (15) has reported recently on his research regarding the quality of the relationship between therapist and patient. He suggests that the importance of the relationship or alliance for the outcome of therapy can be surmised from the fact that research does not support that outcome is strongly influenced by the type of treatment, the characteristics of therapist or patient, or the patient-therapist characteristics matched prior to treatment. His data suggest that an alliance in which the patient experiences the therapist as both helpful and supportive early in treatment is more apt to be noted in patients who improve. A collaborative alliance with emphasis on shared responsibility and a quality of "we-ness" was noted in only a few of the improved patients' relationships with their therapists. Luborsky's findings, however, may be biased in favor of the supportive and against the collaborative alliance by his inclusion of rapport or empathy (a variable of presumed strength) only in the definition of the supportive alliance. Regardless of this question, it is exciting to note the research focus on the nature of the therapeutic relationship.

The collaborative approach to the patient-therapist relationship with its shared power increases the need for contextual clarity. The study of healthy families reveals that there is no confusion about roles. Parents are clearly parents, and yet they are not authoritarian in dealing with children. The roles of therapist and patient need to be clearly distinguished and are seen as complementary. The patient brings to the relationship a variety of problems, enough pain to want to change, and, at the minimum, the potential for trust. The therapist brings a certain body of knowledge and skill, a respect for the patient's individuality, and a commitment to the patient's right to establish his own goals. The nature of the contract between the two must be clear. Although they will be involved in a process which is collaborative and in which intimacy may evolve, their relationship is established in order to help the patient change and grow. The therapist may (and should) learn much about himself or herself, but that learning is not the central purpose of the relationship. That which each participant may expect from the other is explicit.

In addition to the issues of power and clarity, the study of optimal family systems provides the beginning therapist with another framework with which to understand his therapeutic activity. The therapist must develop the capacity to be aware of the characteristics of the human system in which he or she is a participant. This means that the therapist, in addition to being sensitive to the verbal and nonverbal signals from the patient and aware of his or her own thoughts, affects, and fantasies, must develop a sensitivity to the interactional pattern he or she and the patient establish. Awareness of the process of interaction can be taught by focusing the resident's attention upon three interactional variables: the cadence of the interview, the depth of the exploration, and the degree of interpersonal distance or closeness involved in the interaction.

A very troublesome question for the teacher of beginning therapists remains, "what to teach?" One could select and teach a single approach as purely as possible—the practice of psychoanalytic psychotherapy, for example. Another answer would be to attempt to teach all approaches in at least some preliminary way. This presumes the teacher is equally proficient with all approaches or that four different experts are available. Neither of these possibilities is apt to be present in the current reality of training programs. A third approach is to introduce the beginning student to techniques of each of the schools and let him begin to experience the results of their use. When the student understands the origin and theory behind each technique and evolves a synthesis that suits his or her particular temperament, then the teacher may attempt to encourage the concept that variations in technique are called for by the nature of the patient and his or her difficulty. That is the format of the seminar. I agree with the ideal of Havens' call for a pluralistic psychiatry, but feel that providing beginners with attainable goals is one way to give them a headstart on the difficult road to psychotherapeutic competence.

In the seminar to be described, beginning therapists study and practice aspects of therapy that are derived from five different sources. From the objective-descriptive school of psychiatry, the student learns about astute observation of the patient, for example, perception of signs of unusual autonomic nervous system activity in the patient, variations in the pattern of the patient's speech, the ability to observe nonverbal messages and, at a more general level, the value of a clinical formulation or an estimate of both the level and the quality of the patient's psychopathology.

From the psychoanalytic approach to psychiatry, the seminar teaches the student to be able to follow the patient's trains of associations, recognize resistances and mechanisms of defense, and recognize "tips of the iceberg"—markers of largely hidden material—that is, points in the interview when there is the suggestion that the patient is dealing with material that is unusually charged or conflicted. In addition, from this school, the techniques of confrontation and interpretation are introduced.

From the interpersonal school of psychiatry, the student learns the importance of an awareness of therapy as an interaction in which her or she is an inevitable participant. Without this ability, a therapist cannot deal with the patient's projections and assumptions in the relationship.

The focus on affect of the existential school of psychiatry is incorporated into the seminar by an emphasis upon the techniques associated with empathy, warmth, respect, therapist's genuineness, and self-disclosure.

From the research with optimal family systems, the seminar teaches the student how power or interpersonal influence and clarity of individual boundaries are expressed in health-producing ways. From this perspective he or she approaches the difficult task of developing an ability to be aware of the nature of an interaction in which he or she is participating.

FOR BETTER OR WORSE

Any training program for psychotherapists must articulate the incompleteness of our knowledge about effective therapy. Although I believe that research about the outcome of psychotherapy (16) demonstrates that a variety of therapies are effective in inducing personality change, the results of psychotherapy process research are inconclusive. Most therapists can report striking successes, but all must face those occasions in which therapy failed. Lumping many "cases" together in studying outcome tends to blur the lessons of either inspiring improvement or dismal failure, for they *average* in a way that covers the differences, and the successful patient's improvement may be hidden by the worsening of those who do not improve. However, the presence of a large number of patients who do improve demonstrates that psychotherapy can be effective. The fact that some patients worsen as a result of psychotherapy may be insufficiently attended in psychotherapy training programs.

It is mandatory that we communicate clearly to trainees that our understanding of the processes responsible for improvement is incomplete. They must learn to understand that, as with any powerful treatment procedure, the outcome can be detrimental to the patient. The dangers of the psychotherapeutic process must be appreciated. As teachers we can share examples of our own failures along with our successes, but it is my impression that this level of openness is rare. When this type of disclosure is common, there is a possibility that beginners can come to recognize early, and report candidly, when therapy is not going well. Knowledge that some patients do not do well (even outstanding therapists fail with some patients) might soften the blow to their self-esteem. To be able to investigate therapy that is faring poorly at an early stage and to focus on the process of the therapeutic interaction rather than assigning blame might minimize denial and projection.

Any discussion of the outcome of therapy—whether it ends well or poorly—inevitably leads to the question of what we mean by "good" or "bad," and takes one into the complex realm of values.

VALUES AND PSYCHOTHERAPY

In my training some years ago, this area was not addressed, and I labored with the notion that since science was presumed to be value-free, and medicine and psychiatry were certainly "scientific," they were, therefore, independent of considerations of good or bad. Although I was naive, I suspect that others in my generation held similar illusions. Since our generation now staffs the faculty of training programs, perhaps we can introduce our trainees to a deeper understanding of the interface between values and psychotherapy than most of us received.

This psychotherapy seminar presents the view that no psychotherapy is value-free, that each therapist has a group of basic values that are at the center of his or her life, and that they influence all perceptions and each moment of therapy. A therapist can deal with them rationally only by keeping them "up front" in his mind. To be unaware of their existence and potential impact upon patients is to invite their influence in subtle and subterranean ways. There is a question as to whether the therapist's mere awareness of his or her values is enough to preclude their potentially distorting impact. Halleck (17) takes a strong stand and is an eloquent spokesman for those who feel that the therapist must do more than be aware. He is concerned about the power of the therapist's values to influence the patient in a variety of ways. For example, if the psychotherapeutic work focuses only on intrapsychic conflict, the therapist may miss or avoid very real dysfunction in the social system in which the patient participates. Therapy with such a narrow focus may have impact upon the distribution of power within those social systems. It is in the psychiatrist's definition of normality, however, that the greatest opportunity for harm exists. Actually, the therapist's standards may be influenced strongly by conventional value systems, but often the patient may assume mistakenly that they are based solely on scientific facts. Halleck emphasizes that the only protection a patient has is knowledge of what kind of therapeutic outcome the therapist would welcome. As a consequence of this belief, Halleck acquaints his patients with his views on social issues before they start therapy.

Halleck deplores the absence of clear statements within the profession about the value systems because they guide and regulate what he calls the "politics" of psychotherapy. His own position is that values that are central to psychotherapy concern the therapist's views of man's need for intimacy, social power, freedom, openness to experience, action, privacy, hope, stability, non-violence, and a sense of personal meaning.

In introducing beginning therapists to the impact of their own values upon their psychotherapy transactions, we explore personal answers to several fundamental questions. The first is, "What is the nature of man?" Psychiatric residents and psychology graduate students, in particular, tend to have a mind-set based upon biology or observation and experimentation with animals. Eisenberg's essay (18) on the human nature of human nature discloses the inadequate foundation in fact of those who would extrapolate directly from animal to man, and discusses the tremendous impact of language and culture on human behavior. This is not, however, only a theoretical issue. Eisenberg (p. 123) states:

> What we believe of man affects the behavior of men, for it determines what each expects of the other. Theories of education, of political science, of economics, and the very policies of governments are based on implicit concepts of the nature of man. Is he educable? Is he a creature of such dark lusts that only submission to sovereign authority can save him from himself?

Each therapist must ponder these issues and have a personal answer to the question, "What is the nature of man?" The seminar does not hold the answer. Rather, it raises the question and emphasizes that the therapist can never evade or escape the impact of this answer on his or her patients.

The second fundamental question is, "What is the meaning of life?" Here, too, the beginning therapist needs to evolve a clear position. Many patients will be seen who cling to a life situation that is inimical to what the therapist feels life is all about. How do the therapist's values regarding the meaning of life influence his or her responses to such a patient? Should the therapist's own values influence the treatment goals of the patient? Once again, clarity and awareness on the part of the therapist regarding the issues are crucial.

It has been helpful to introduce the students to Spiegel and Kluckhohn's (19) format for assessing the relativity of cultural value orientations. These authors suggest that each culture (and, I would add, each sub-culture) suggests an answer to four basic questions: 1) What is the relation of man to nature? 2) What is the temporal focus of human life? 3) What is the ideal human activity? 4) What is the optimal form of man's relationships with other men? Western culture—despite rapid change—continues to teach that man is the master of nature, primarily concerned about the future rather than the past or present, more significantly involved with "doing" than "being," and highly individualistic in relationships with other men.

The seminar introduces the student to the complexities of the effect of values on psychotherapy. It suggests that, at the minimum, a therapist must be clear about his or her values and mindful of their impact on therapeutic relationships. This need for awareness raises the issue of the nature of the relationship he or she strives for with patients.

THE BALANCE OF INTIMACY AND DETACHMENT

Of all the skills to be acquired by the beginning therapist, the balance of intimacy and detachment with patients is perhaps the most difficult. There are few guidelines, and in spite of its importance, few training programs attend the issue directly. The sensitive, experienced therapist constantly monitors this balance with each patient, and the fluctuations he or she perceives are used as important sources of understanding the process of the ongoing therapy. A goal of the seminar is for the beginning therapist to be able to recognize both the intimacy and the detachment he or she experiences with patients, and to be sensitive to variations in the balance between the two.

The problem of finding an appropriate balance of intimacy

and detachment is not restricted to psychotherapists, but troubles all the helping professions. Training to be a professional provides one with a body of knowledge and skills to be offered to others as a professional service. This must be done in a way that requires the professional to perceive the patient and his problems objectively. To do so requires a degree of interpersonal distance and a particular way of perceiving the patient, who is seen as the bearer of symptoms rather than as a whole person. The helper focuses attention on symptoms, signs, associations, projective maneuvers, or other "part aspects" of the patient, at times detaching himself or herself even further in order to put together the observations, consider correlations, synthesize, and from this, construct hypotheses about the patient. The therapist must choose whether or not to intervene and, if so, the nature of the intervention to be used. During these periods, the activity of the therapist is primarily cognitive—observing, thinking, analyzing, hypothesizing. All of these cognitive activities require considerable detachment and emotional distance from the patient.

In addition, however, a psychotherapist is "with" the patient in a different kind of way. The therapist either allows himself to be drawn into the patient's affective world, or more actively pursues this type of affective sharing. During these moments in therapy, the therapist suspends his or her more analytic and detached cognitive processes and feels whatever the patient seems to be feeling. This involves a process of "letting go." At such times, the interpersonal distance between patient and therapist is markedly reduced. This type of activity by the therapist permits him to be *with* the patient in a different way and to experience something of what the patient is feeling. Additionally, however, it allows the therapist's own memories and fantasies to emerge into consciousness, which may be the source of further understanding of the patient. This way of relating is called, more often than not, empathy and is the subject of Chapter 2.

These two basic ways of relating to another person are so different that to master them concurrently is a difficult and complicated task. A desirable balance is a flexible one in which the therapist moves back and forth between the two activities. This task is made difficult by a number of factors. First, each of the various schools of psychiatry suggests its own bias about the optimal balance. The objective-descriptive school dictates a balance heavily weighted in the direction of detachment in which the therapist is, at his or her core, an "objective observer" interested in as precise an understanding as possible of the symptoms and signs of the patient's illness. Although he or she may be a warm and interested professional, such a model of the patient's difficulty does not suggest that the empathic process is central to understanding and helping.

As an aside, I would suggest that any professional, of whatever discipline, who is dominated by a narrowly defined model of disease and who has an objective-descriptive manner of relating to patients, runs the risk of being perceived by the patients as interested only in their disease and not at all in their welfare as a whole person. The exciting advances of molecular biology have moved medicine in general to this position, and it is not surprising that patients frequently complain that the doctor does not listen and seems interested only in the disease and the laboratory findings. Within psychiatry, for example, the recent advances in understanding neurobiological processes, coupled with the attempt to understand psychiatric disturbances primarily in terms of neurotransmitter chemistry, have led to a resurgence of the objective-descriptive style of relating to patients. In psychology, the emergence of behavior modification and biofeedback has pushed the balance of intimacy and detachment in the direction of detachment. Perhaps the development of an increasingly precise technology in any discipline moves its practitioners in the direction of increased interpersonal distance from patients.

The psychoanalytic school of psychiatry is, at its heart, an objective approach that emphasizes the neutral position of the therapist. The psychoanalytic therapist monitors the patient's associations sensitively and, although subscribing to the importance of empathy, emphasizes the role of interpretation. There are exceptions to this generalization, and the writings of Greenson (20), Schafer, (21), and Paul (22) are examples of a growing emphasis upon the importance of the therapist's empathic work.

The interpersonal school can also be seen as emphasizing a balance in the direction of detachment. The therapist is an active, confronting agent primarily concerned with the patient's assumptions and distortions. As a consequence, the therapist is interested in clarifying interpersonal reality. In counterprojective maneuvers, the therapist does not hesitate to be overtly manipulative. Although relying upon empathic processes to understand the patient's distorting assumptions, the balance is weighted in the direction of detachment. The therapist's expertise is concerned centrally with the ability to undo the patient's projections objectively in the here-and-now of their interaction.

The existential school does not espouse a balance of intimacy and detachment, for all objectivity is seen as interfering with being and staying. Analyzing, synthesizing, and concluding are to be avoided, as they are symptomatic of the therapist's defeat by the patient's efforts to avoid the pain of intimacy. This school of psychotherapy calls for a total subjectivity in a way similar to the objective-descriptive school's mandate for nearly total detachment. The psychoanalytic and interpersonal schools are midway between these extremes, and both emphasize the importance of empathic processes, although the balance favors the therapist's ability to analyze and interpret or to move actively against projections.

Two of the major approaches to psychotherapy appear to require no balance, but rely upon either intimacy or detachment. The other two schools, although varying with the writer, suggest a mixture in which the therapist's capacity for therapeutic work is weighted in the direction of detachment. This rather fundamental disagreement among schools leads to confusion for a beginner. He or she is often influenced by the stance of one or another teacher who may neglect to emphasize the fact that experts do not agree and that research does not substantiate the value of one approach over another.

A second source of difficulty for beginners is the likelihood that whatever native capacity for intimacy they possessed may have been washed out by the process of their education. They come to a psychiatric residency after eight years of careful training in detachment. The competitive struggle of undergraduate premedical education is won most easily by students who mobilize a compulsive adaptation. Knowing facts, analyzing cognitive problems, and synthesizing details augment one's chances for admission to medical school. Medical education is dominated by the advances in molecular biology, and usually disease is defined solely in terms of cellular processes. The patient as a whole person is too often overlooked in the rush to define disease precisely. The medical student often is taught little in any systematic way about the patient's subjective experience of illness. Underneath all of this, the message to the student is all on the side of detachment. The teacher or bedside clinician with the more detached skills *and* empathic capabilities is less available as an identification model. The price of wonderful, technical advances has too often been diminished humanism.

It is likely that medical education not only rewards detachment, but selects its students on that basis. Cassell (23) has described the "healing connection" and, despite the task of operationalizing the concept, there is little to suggest great interest on the part of medical school admissions committees and faculties.

The educational process has a similar impact in graduate education in psychology and social work. It appears that students of all disciplines come to their training in psychotherapy with a heavy bias in the direction of objectivity and detachment. Early clinical experiences further confuse them. They find that patients have different impacts. Some push towards extreme detachment; others pull toward an intimacy that may frighten. How often the students may find that work with an obsessive patient results in interview after interview of sterile ruminations or that work with a hysteric patient involves a sense of closeness associated with intense affective arousal. In addition to the complexity of these factors in themselves, supervisors help the students to appreciate that their own capacity to achieve a helpful balance between intimacy and detachment varies from day to day or week to week. The students come to learn that an illness in a spouse may move him or her to an entrenched detachment, or a spouse's prolonged absence may make closeness with patients more attractive.

To balance intimacy and detachment is a difficult and never-ending struggle. For most beginning therapists, detachment is familiar and safe. Intimacy, particularly with the kind of discipline required of the therapist, may seem both unfamiliar and dangerous. The initial task of the teacher is to introduce the concept that a balance is required and, through a variety of exercises, provide the student with opportunities to experience the unfamiliar and to tolerate and learn this type of disciplined intimacy. It is within this context that the seminar begins to study and practice the principles of empathy.

REFERENCES

1. CHESSICK, R. D., *How Psychotherapy Heals.* New York: Science House, 1969.
2. CHESSICK, R. D., *Why Psychotherapists Fail.* New York: Science House, 1971.
3. MATARAZZO, R. G., WIENS, A. N., and SASLOW, G., "Experimentation in the Teaching and Learning of Psychotherapy Skills." In: A. Gottschalk, and A. H. Auerbach (eds.), *Methods of Research in Psychotherapy.* New York: Appleton-Century-Crofts, 1966, p. 608.
4. NAMNUM, A., "Activity and Personal Involvement in Psychoanalytic Technique." *Bulletin of the Menninger Clinic,* Vol. 40:2, 105-117, March, 1976.
5. ROGERS, C. R., *The Therapeutic Relationship and Its Impact: A Study of Psychotherapy with Schizophrenics.* Madison, Milwaukee, and London: The University of Wisconsin Press, 1967.
6. TRUAX, C. B., and CARKHUFF, R. R., *Toward Effective Counseling and Psychotherapy: Training and Practice.* New York: Aldine, 1967.
7. CARKHUFF, R. R., *Helping and Human Relations,* Vol. I & II. New York: Holt, Rinehart & Winston, Inc., 1969.
8. LEWIS, J. M., BEAVERS, W. R., GOSSETT, J. T., and PHILLIPS, V. A., *No Single Thread: Psychological Health in Family Systems.* New York: Brunner/Mazel, 1976.
9. BEAVERS, W. R., *Psychotherapy and Growth: A Family Systems Perspective.* New York: Brunner/Mazel, 1977.
10. BROMBERG, W., *Man Above Humanity.* Philadelphia: J. B. Lippincott, 1954.
11. FRANK, J. D., *Persuasion and Healing.* Baltimore and London: The Johns Hopkins University Press, 1973.
12. HAVENS, L. L., "The Existential Use of the Self." *American Journal of Psychiatry,* 131:1, 1-10, January, 1974.
13. HAVENS, L. L., *Approaches to the Mind.* Boston: Little, Brown and Company, 1973.

14. HAVENS, L. L., *Participant Observation.* New York: Jason Aronson, Inc., 1976.
15. LUBORSKY, L., "Helping Alliances in Psychotherapy." In: J. L. Claghorn (ed.), *Successful Psychotherapy.* New York: Brunner/Mazel, 1976.
16. MELTZOFF, J., and KORNREICH, M., *Research in Psychotherapy.* New York: Atherton Press, Inc., 1970.
17. HALLECK, S. L., *The Politics of Therapy.* New York: Science House, Inc., 1971.
18. EISENBERG, L., "The Human Nature of Human Nature." *Science,* 176:4031, pp. 123-128, April 14, 1972.
19. SPIEGEL, J. P., and KLUCKHOHN, F. In: J. Spiegel, *Transactions: The Interplay Between Individual, Family, and Society.* New York: Science House, 1971, p. 163.
20. GREENSON, R. R., "Empathy and Its Vicissitudes." *International Journal of Psychoanalysis,* 41:418-424, 1960.
21. SCHAFER, R., "Generative Empathy in the Treatment Situation." *The Psychoanalytic Quarterly,* 28:3, 342-371, 1959.
22. PAUL, N. L., "The Use of Empathy in the Resolution of Grief." *Perspectives in Biology and Medicine,* Vol. 11, pp. 153-169, 1967-68.
23. CASSELL, E. J., *The Healer's Art.* Philadelphia: J. B. Lippincott Company, 1976.

CHAPTER 2

+++

Empathy

+++

++

Achieving a balance between intimacy and detachment requires
that the beginning therapist be capable of a particular kind of
intimacy. It implies a sharing of the patient's inmost self with the
discipline necessary to pull back to a position of detachment—
indeed, to alternate states of intimacy and detachment during the
course of each psychotherapy session. It is closeness that is primarily for the patient regardless of how it is experienced by the
therapist; this, too, requires discipline. In addition, the experienced therapist monitors the changing balance of intimacy and
detachment throughout each session, and this also requires a disciplined awareness. Although I stress the disciplined aspect of the
intimacy required of the therapist, the problem most often presented by the beginning therapist is an inability to release the
hold on his or her feelings and achieve periods of intimacy with
the patient. Learning the techniques of empathy in a structured
way provides the student with a graduated experience in intimacy.

Empathy is concerned primarily with understanding feelings. The importance of affectivity has not had a central place in recent psychodynamic formulations. Although early psychoanalytic formulations included terms of affectivity, the focus gradually changed to emphasize more clearly genetic, dynamic, and structural viewpoints. Isaacs and Haggard (1) suggest a recent resurgence of interest in affect, and their research documents its central position in the technique of psychotherapy. They demonstrate that patient statements of high levels of meaning were more apt to follow therapists' statements containing affect words. Therapists' use of affect words differed widely. (The range was from 1½% to 77% of therapists' statements.) They suggest that, regardless of therapists' theoretical orientations, those therapists who respond to patients' affect are more likely to elicit meaningful responses from patients. It is this attention to patients' affect that is vitally connected to the ability to be empathic.

Psychotherapists generally agree that empathy is important, but they vary greatly in the way they define the term. Existential psychiatrists (2), more than adherents of other schools, consider empathy a central skill. Their key concept is that of "being with" —the attempt by the therapist to place himself or herself where the patient is emotionally. It includes both understanding and feeling close. The therapist tries to stay with the patient without any attempt to confirm prior hypotheses. Indeed, the therapist must avoid cognitive conclusions. The therapist's activity, literally projecting himself or herself into the patient's feeling world, is the major objective of empathy. Although translating, self-disclosure, and confrontation are also important techniques in this approach, its focus is on feelings and the therapist's capacity to *be* and *stay* where the patient is emotionally. Thus, this existential definition of empathy emphasizes the therapist's own capacity to feel.

Psychoanalytic writers (3, 4) have defined empathy in a similar way. The capacity of the therapist to feel that which the patient feels is described by them as a temporary regression of the ego in the service of the psychotherapeutic process. The difference between the psychoanalytic concept of empathy and that of the existentialists has more to do with the goals of empathy than with the process itself. Psychoanalytic writers emphasize the ability of the therapist to move back and forth from empathy to a more objective analysis (rather than being and staying emotionally with the patient as an objective in itself). Despite these differences, both psychoanalysts and existentialists define empathy primarily in terms of the therapist's capacity to be aroused. This type of empathy may be termed "affective empathy" (5) or "compathy"(6).

Rogers and his followers (7, 8, 9) have done research in the role of empathy in psychotherapy. Their definition of empathy emphasizes the capacity of the therapist both to perceive accurately what the patient is feeling and to communicate this awareness to the patient. This definition of empathy relates more to the therapist's perceptual and communication skills than to the degree of his or her own affective arousal. The empathy scales of these writers emphasize the sensitivity of the therapist to the patient's affect rather than the feelings of the therapist. This type of empathy may be termed "cognitive empathy."

Bachrach (10) has reviewed the research about the role of empathy in the outcome of psychotherapy, and he argues cogently that what is measured in such research may not be identical with empathy as defined in clinical theory. His particular focus is on empathy as a "kind of attitude or way of perceiving" that the therapist assumes, rather than something he says or does.

Orlinsky and Howard (11) present research data to suggest that the therapist's "empathic induction" is more apt to agree with the patient's self-reports than is the therapist's objective perception. Empathic induction is defined as a feeling the therapist gets in the patient's presence. The feeling may be experienced as free-floating or elaborated as a fantasy. The feeling is said to result from a sensori-motor accommodation to subtle changes in the patient's expressive behavior. There is, however, no self-evident sensory reference. This ability of the therapist is based upon responsiveness, sensitivity, and the capacity of take into account his or her own idiosyncratic tendencies. These authors emphasize the necessity for the therapist to keep in touch with both his or her own and the patient's experience in order to make the "vital connection" that permits therapy to occur. This definition of empathy focuses on the therapist's feeling state as responsive to subtle messages from the patient and, as such, it is related to both affective and cognitive empathy.

Muslin (12), a student and teacher of psychotherapy, has defined the empathic process carefully. He sees the special nature of the process as derived from the prior experiences of the therapist. He describes the initial stage of being empathic as an observation of the psychological state of the patient that is sufficient to stimulate memory traces in the therapist of his or her previously experienced psychological states. This perception and arousal phase is followed by the therapist's self-observations. The therapist then uses these memories, thoughts, feelings, and sensations as a basis for the appreciation of the patient's mental state. Muslin emphasizes the difference between this type of empathic process and the total subjective reaction of the therapist precipitated by the patient.

Although Muslin's operational definition of the empathic process includes both an initial perceptual phase and the arousal of the therapist's affect, and is, I believe, a most careful conceptualization of the process, I wish to emphasize the advantages of conceptualizing empathy as a continuum along which two factors are present to varying degrees: the interpersonal distance between therapist and patient and the degree of the therapist's affective arousal.

Cognitive empathy can be described as the capacity of the therapist to perceive the manifest feelings of the patient accurately. There is little arousal of therapist's affect, and there is considerable interpersonal distance between therapist and patient. Affective empathy is described as the feelings aroused in the therapist as he or she strives to be with the patient emotionally. The therapist's affect is aroused, and the interpersonal distance between therapist and patient is reduced. My experience with this seminar suggests that it is important to start teaching the techniques at the level of cognitive empathy as this is a learning exercise with more readily attainable goals.

Many therapists have available to them the full range of empathy. My experience as a therapist is that during empathic periods (that is, when not observing, analyzing, and synthesizing), I am usually nearer the cognitive empathy end of the continuum. I try to attend the patient's moment-to-moment affective messages and, in so doing, am not particularly caught up in my own affective state. Periodically, however, one of several things may occur. I may either move actively into the affective state the patient is experiencing or, without any sense of action or moving out to the patient's affect, simply come to feel the affect or experience a charged fantasy or memory. Occasionally, I note that a period of cognitive empathy is followed by evidence of my own anxiety in the form of boredom or irritation (for me, presumptive evidence of anxiety). At such times, it seems particularly important to allow or encourage the emergence (to myself) of my own affect. An example may clarify this change in level of empathy.

The patient, a 36-year-old man, was seen three times a week over a period of several years. Diagnostically he was seen as a severe borderline syndrome with multiple addictions. Periodically, he regressed to a very helpless and clinging position. On some occasions these regressions necessitated hospitalization. During the third year of psychotherapy, he appeared again to be moving in the direction of helplessness. Before the interview from which the following excerpt is taken I found myself anxious about the possible need for another period of hospitalization and increasingly doubtful about the effectiveness of our work together.

Patient: . . . I . . . can't go on . . . I can't do anything . . . someone must take care of me.
Therapist: You're feeling helpless . . . can't continue on your own.
Patient: (crying) . . . I . . . put me in the hospital . . . do something.
Therapist: You want me to take over—take care of you?
Patient: (sobs for several minutes)

At this point, I felt anxious and uncertain—wondering if I should assume a more authoritarian role and admit him to a hospital. I felt also some irritation and made an active effort to get more in touch with myself. Quickly a memory came to mind of awakening from anesthesia following a surgical procedure at age seven. I felt again the sick, helpless feeling, and the tremendous sense of aloneness that went with it. It was a painful memory and gave me a much clearer sense of what my patient might be experiencing. In particular, the sense of aloneness I reexperienced in my early memory was, I thought, an aspect of the patient's current state that I was not in touch with as my concern about his helplessness and my response to it had dominated my own reaction.

Therapist: A . . . I get the feeling that as part of it . . . a big part of it . . . a big part of where you are right now . . . the feeling of being alone.

Patient: . . . (quietly) yea . . . that's so much of it . . . alone . . . I always end up feeling alone . . . even here with you I . . . it's like I'm alone . . . not all the time . . . but when it's like this . . . it's so alone.

This level of affective empathy was not only helpful in my understanding of the patient's experience, but enabled us to reinstitute a working relationship in which his profound sense of aloneness could be explored.

There is another approach to describing empathy, and that is as a characteristic of an interaction between two or more individuals. According to this position, it is not something an individual either has or does not have, but rather a dimension of an ongoing relationship. There are, for example, a few psychophysiologic experiments that suggest that empathy can be studied usefully as an interactional process. Charny (13), in his slow-motion photographic study of a doctor-patient interview, noted the presence of very rapid total body vibrations of small amplitude that are undetectable to the naked eye. Utilizing the slow-motion camera, he found that at moments judged by observers to be of high rapport, the doctor's and the patient's vibrations became synchronous. In another study, DiMascio and co-workers (14) noted that, during periods of high rapport during a psychotherapy interview, there was a curious parallelism between the patient's and the therapist's pulse rates that was not noted during periods of lesser rapport. These findings, although obviously requiring more study and replication, suggest a physiological basis for the poetic phrase, "two hearts that beat as one."

It may be that any schema that approaches empathy as a therapist's characteristic, skill, or attribute misses the mark by grossly underestimating the interactional complexity of the phenomenon. Nevertheless, viewing empathy as a quality of an individual (the therapist) has value for training.

THE FUNCTIONS OF EMPATHY

Empathy has several major functions in effective psychotherapy. The first is the creation of moments when the patient feels that a significant other is deeply with him and that he is truly understood. This experience is considered by some to be, in itself, an important factor in the emotional growth of the patient. Havens (2) has emphasized its relevance for the existential therapy constructs of "being" and "staying." Such moments are the aim of treatment and felt to be curative. Strupp (15) has pointed out that some years after successful therapy, patients often point to their therapist's deep understanding as one of the helpful aspects of treatment. The Rogerian writers (9) present research findings that high levels of therapist (cognitive) empathy are correlated significantly with patient improvement. Chessick (16, 17) emphasizes the role of the therapist in presenting the patient with ideal conditions for psychotherapy, and includes empathy as an important vector. It appears, therefore, that students of psychotherapy from diverse schools accept, to one degree or another, that the therapist's empathy plays an important role in the patient's change and growth.

A second function of empathy is that of facilitating self-exploration. Whether one accepts the idea that empathy has some curative or growth-inducing value, research has shown that patients who feel that their therapist understands their feelings precisely are induced to share more of themselves. It has been my observation that high levels of therapist cognitive empathy

result in a greater degree of patient self-exploration. Unless a
therapist is dealing with a patient who has major or profound
resistances to the exploration of affect (and, of course, there are
such patients), a consistently high level of empathic responsiveness to the patient's affective messages leads to increasing exploration on the part of the patient.

A third function of empathy involves the therapist's understanding of the patient. This may occur in a number of ways.
The therapist may note, for example, the apparent absence of
affect at times when the patient is describing a life circumstance
or memory that would seem to carry considerable feelings with
it for most persons. The therapist may project himself or herself
into the patient's life circumstance and, momentarily, "let go" of
his or her own feelings silently. The therapist, by the use of this
empathic capacity, has encountered what may be the patient's
resistance in the form of denial. Something of value has been
learned about the patient. The patient, for example, may be
describing the death of a parent. There is no apparent affect. The
therapist allows a significant personal loss to be reexperienced,
feels the sadness, and begins to construct a very tentative hypothesis: The affect surrounding the death of the parent may be too
painful for the patient to experience directly with the therapist
at this time.

These three goals or functions of empathy are often operating
at the same time; they are not mutually exclusive. The therapist,
at a given moment of empathic responsiveness, may be offering
the patient ingredients basic to all helpful relationships—encouraging the patient to deeper self-exploration and gathering data
that help the therapist to understand the patient's psychopathology more accurately. Small wonder that diverse approaches to
psychotherapy suggest that a high level of therapist's empathy
is crucial to effective psychotherapy!

RESISTANCES TO EMPATHY

Beginning therapists demonstrate widely differing empathic
capacities. Although some are much more sensitive to affective

messages than others, very few reveal much in the way of affective empathy. As noted in Chapter 1, this may reflect both the criteria used in selecting medical and graduate students and the intense emphasis upon "objectivity" experienced by the students during their years of education. Students' feelings about patients are often considered an unwelcome intrusion, with no diagnostic or therapeutic value.

It has been suggested (18) that an individual's empathic capacity starts developing after numerous empathic experiences as an infant with his or her mother. Our own research with families indicates that families of widely different competencies can be distinguished from each other by a combination of ten or twelve variables. One of these family variables is the level of family empathy. Some families not only express more feelings, but respond to each other's feelings with high levels of empathy. There are no comprehensive research data regarding the families of origin of mental health professionals, but the suggestion has been made (19) that, as a group, their families of origin may be skewed towards the pathological. If this is so, there are many exceptions to the generalization. These ideas about mother-infant interactions and the level of empathy in one's family of origin as determinants of the adult level of empathy are interesting but, at the present time, we have little data about the development over time of empathy. At an impressionistic level, one can observe that students who isolate their own affect and relate to others distantly have greater difficulty learning the techniques of empathy.

Muslin and Schlessinger (20) have reported their experiences in teaching empathy to psychiatric residents and present in considerable detail observations about the reactions to, and interferences with, the empathic process. They describe two distorting modes of observation. The first, "pathologizing," based on the "medical model," stresses objectivity and avoids introspection. In part, pathologizing is furthered by early work with inpatients with serious ego defects, which they continue to see in patients who present no actual evidence of such defects. The authors indicate that the process of pathologizing may represent an attempt to increase distance from patients by emphasizing the differences between therapists and patients. In reviewing videotapes of interviews in which the resident observers had pathologized the patient, it was often instructive to elicit the fantasies of the residents about the patient. In this way, clues as to the use of pathologizing were often uncovered.

The second observational mode used as resistance to the empathic process is termed "normalizing." Here the residents attempt to minimize overt pathology. Often, the residents responded to such patients as if they were normal people who had only been victimized by oppressive social forces (at times, of course, this was true). To "normalize" may reflect a need of the trainee to deny pathology on the basis that responding empathically to the pathological affect would produce significant anxiety for the trainee.

Muslin and Schlessinger also describe defenses and affects that interfere with empathic observations. They use as an example the attractive patient who stimulates sexual feelings in the trainee. This affect, then, interferes with the capacity for empathy. Any affect that produces discomfort in the trainee can reduce the capacity for empathy.

Some students respond to personally distressing feelings stimulated by a patient by projecting that affect to the patient. For example, a trainee who is angered by the patient's passivity can mistakenly think that the patient is angry. Intellectualization and transient identifications with the patient may be used as resistances to empathy rather than in the service of understanding the patient.

Katz (21) has also discussed at length difficulties with the empathic process. He cites a natural decline in empathic powers as the maturing therapist becomes increasingly vulnerable to stereotypes and conventions. Many errors in empathizing are related to personal anxieties of the therapist which may move him or her toward either overidentification or excessive distance. A major problem for those who are able to be empathic is projecting themselves into the world of another and then neglecting to respect the integrity and separateness of the other.

Katz categorizes therapists who do not empathize effectively
into five groups: 1) the "marginal" empathizer, who penetrates
only a part of the patient's experience; 2) the "evangelical"
therapist who is so concerned with changing the patient that he
or she fails to empathize effectively; 3) the "hysteric" empathizer
who overidentifies in a symbiotic way; 4) the "compulsive" empathizer who can identify with one ego state of the patient, but
cannot easily shift this identification; and 5) the "rationalistic"
empathizer who cannot abandon his or her professional role and
underidentifies with the patient.

In order to treat patients empathically, the private life of the
therapist must have "a dignity of its own, offering personal gratification . . ." If the therapist must use the therapeutic situation
to compensate for poverty of personal life, the therapist is apt to
take from rather than give to the patient.

The difficulties I have encountered in teaching empathy relate
directly to those described in the above literature. The most common problem encountered is the intellectually gifted, but significantly obsessive, beginner who is unable to have free access
to personal feelings and to "let go." The skills of cognitive empathy may be learned, but affective empathy is unattainable. Less
frequently, a beginner with no problem letting go will experience
difficulty in "coming back." An impressive capacity for interpersonal closeness and affective arousal is not matched with the
discipline required to return to a position of greater distance and
increased objectivity. Also, I would emphasize that the student
needs a psychosocial network that provides the opportunity for
satisfying intimacy, in order that it not be searched for inappro-
priately with patients.

Ten years of experience with this approach to training for first-
year residents and other mental health professionals, leads me to
the following conclusions:

1) Cognitive empathy is easily teachable to most beginning
therapists.

2) Affective empathy is a process to which a teacher can only
introduce the trainee. It is not easily taught, but depends upon

the level of ego functioning of the trainee. For some trainees, the freedom to "let go" or the discipline required to "come back" is so counter to their personality structure that intensive personal therapy may be required to alter such limitations. Affective empathy can be taught to beginning therapists who enter training with healthy levels of ego functioning, but even here is not *easily* learned.

3) The capacity for affective empathy may be the essence of that which separates the competent from the gifted therapists. However, it is indispensable in the successful psychotherapeutic treatment of the severely disturbed patient. Whether the patient is psychotic or severely borderline, the chances for successful outcome are augmented significantly if the therapist is able to experience something of his or her own infantile core.

EMPATHY TRAINING

The seminar is taught to seven to ten students each year. At the start, they are introduced to two different styles of interviewing: directive interviewing and collaborative exploration. Frequently the only method of interviewing they know is directive interviewing, in which the therapist asks questions and the patient answers the questions. The interviewer selects and controls the direction of the interview (although influenced by the patient's answers). The therapist is clearly the expert and may focus on the patient's symptoms, fantasies, or feelings. This type of interview maximizes the power differential between the two and is characteristic of history-taking in medicine, the objective-descriptive school of psychiatry, and most dialogues involving an expert in any field with a patient or client.

On the other hand, collaborative exploration is a different technique in which the interviewer minimizes the amount of direct and focused questioning and encourages the patient to explore problems. The therapist does so by general requests such as "tell me more" or "please go on." The therapist also reflects, summarizes, and responds empathically. This style of interviewing is collaborative because the interviewer wants the direction of the dialogue to come from the patient and, in that sense, there is a sharing of power. This type of interview format is characteristic of both the psychoanalytic and existential schools of psychiatry. A brief example of each interviewing format is presented for clarification.

Directive Interviewing

> *Therapist*: Can you tell me what seems to be the problem?
> *Patient*: I don't know exactly . . . it's a feeling of anxiety . . . as if something bad is going to happen.
> *Therapist*: When did you first notice it?
> *Patient*: About three months ago.
> *Therapist*: Did it start suddenly?
> *Patient*: Yes—I just woke up one morning feeling that way.
> *Therapist*: What was going on in your life at that time?
> *Patient*: Nothing in particular.
> *Therapist*: Were you under any unusual stress?
> *Patient*: Not that I know of . . .
> *Therapist*: At work or at home with your family?
> *Patient*: No—everything seemed to be fine.
> *Therapist*: Has the anxious feeling been constant during the three months?
> *Patient*: No—at times I feel normal.
> *Therapist*: What are the circumstances that seem to make the difference?
> *Patient*: I don't know, I can't tell—it just suddenly leaves me.

Collaborative Interviewing

> *Therapist*: Can you tell me how you've been feeling?
> *Patient*: It's hard to describe—sort of a feeling of anxiety —as if something bad is going to happen.
> *Therapist*: Anxious, something bad about to happen?
> *Patient*: Yes . . .
> *Therapist*: Help me to understand it more.
> *Patient*: Well—for about three months now—much of the time I just have this terrible feeling—like a sense of doom—and I am aware of my heart beating and my palms sweat.
> *Therapist*: It sounds terribly uncomfortable . . .
> *Patient*: It really is—it's the worse thing I've experienced—

> nothing compares to it . . . I've had some hairy times in
> the service—but I know what that was about . . .
> *Therapist*: Go on . . .
> *Patient*: Well—in the war—there were situations when I
> could have been killed . . . friends—guys in my outfit
> were . . .
> *Therapist*: Does this anxiety have some of that in it? . . .
> *Patient*: What . . .? Well . . . . I think . . . yes. I've never
> really said it—but there is something—a fear—that I
> might die.
> *Therapist*: So . . . the anxious feeling involves death or
> dying . . .
> *Patient*: Yea . . . but—I'm in good health . . . There isn't any
> reason . . . but, yes . . . I do feel that I might die . . .
> that I won't live long enough to see my children grow
> up . . . That's part of it.

The students learn that, more often than not, a collaborative format is most useful in psychotherapeutic interviews, and directive interviewing is more suited to history-taking or a mental status examination.

Following this general introduction, the students turn to a series of structured exercises designed to increase their understanding of cognitive empathy and sensitivity to manifest affective messages from patients. The first exercise consists of 16 audiotaped "patient stimuli" statements taken from Carkhuff's text (9, Vol. I, 100-104). The students are instructed to consider each statement as occurring in an initial or early interview. They are asked to respond in as helpful a way as possible and to write their responses on paper. The 16 statements represent five different content areas (social-interpersonal, educational-vocational, child rearing, sexual-marital, and confrontation of therapist), and each area of content is paired with three different affects (depression-distress, anger-hostility, and elation-excitement). Each student reads his or her response to each stimulus statement aloud, and the instructor and participants comment. Most responses are focused questions requesting more information or giving advice. Usually, the majority respond to the content of the stimulus statement and disregard the affect. When his or her response has been less than helpful, the beginning therapist experiences considerable discomfort in reading the response aloud. The instructor must offer a good deal of tact, and it is helpful to share his or her own errors with students.

A simple formula is offered to the students as an aid in orienting their responses. They are told to listen for both the affect and the content, and to formulate a response that reflects both. It is helpful if the student can attend the content first and end the response with a reflection of the affect. The entire response should have an invitational quality—some implicit request for the patient to proceed.

They are told to listen only for the obvious; "reading in" hidden or "deeper" meaning of affect is discouraged. The goal of the response is only to let the patient know that the therapist has perceived what the patient has said and what the patient is feeling.

It is helpful for the students to have some measure with which to evaluate responses, both their own and those of their colleagues. An informal, four-level scale is provided. An interchangeable or same-level response is one that reflects back accurately both the content and manifest affect contained in the stimulus statement. A "reach" is a response that is accurate at an interchangeable level but tries to do a little more, to reach a deeper level of the patient's experience. A "take away" is a response that reflects the content and quality of affect accurately but minimizes the intensity of the affect (when a patient's rage is labeled irritation, for example). An "out of the room" response is one that has so little relationship to the stimulus that it is difficult to know that the therapist was in the same room with the patient.

When each student's response to each of the 16 statements has been read and discussed, a second set of audiotaped stimuli statements is played.* Rather than writing the responses on paper, however, the student responds privately into another tape recorder. There are 90 seconds allowed to respond to each stimulus statement. The 10 statements are more difficult in many ways.

---

* Audiotape created at Timberlawn Foundation.

Some express more intense feelings than the first group. Often the stimulus statement does not explicitly label the affect (as is often true in the first group)—rather, the affect is communicated by tone of voice. The statements are replicated here in order to share their complexity and anxiety-provoking nature.

Stimulus # 1

"My mother hasn't given me a moment's peace in the last three months. Ever since my father died she has depended on me more and more. She's quite old and I'd like to enjoy her in what I feel must be the last few years of her life, but she makes such demands on me that I find myself angry with her most of the time. She has no interests of her own; will not spend any time with her own friends, and then she seems to resent it when I have other things that I want to do— not to mention the responsibilities other than entertaining and taking care of her. Now, if she really were incapable of caring for herself, I'd consider a nursing home for her, but I'm not sure that's the case. I think she simply wants to occupy all my time."

Stimulus # 2

"Yeah, yeah, you always have a suggestion don't you? Everything's clear-cut and simple, just like that. Well, what about you? I hear you're getting a divorce. How can I trust you to help me solve my problems when you can't even solve your own?"

Stimulus # 3

"Oh, goddamn, can't you help me? I don't even want to think about it."

Stimulus # 4

"Well, I had problems, you know, but I never did think anything about them. I guess I just bottled them up. I had, uh, or tried to have a normal family life. You know, I was just a kid, and I played the part of a kid and I'd like to go back to it. I thought it was just great."

Stimulus # 5

"You know, you understand everything I say. You really hear me. My husband has never been like that. I can't seem to make him understand what I want from him. You're the only person in the world who really understands me, but this whole thing is so one-sided. I want to know what you feel too. I want to know if you find me as attractive and appealing as I find you, because if you do, there are other places for us to meet instead of here in this damned office."

Stimulus # 6

"Well, yeah, it's an escape. I've searched and I think my pretense is my hair, cause I like my hair. I mean, I like to have it grow, and grow, and grow, and grow—of course, it isn't now because I keep getting busted and put in jail, and it keeps getting cut, because when I walk down the street, here I am with my long hair. And people, some people would trip me, but then some people put me down and look at me strange. I like that too. Some people wouldn't even spit on me for some reason, you know. In terms, I mean, like they walk away real fast and they don't want to get involved."

Stimulus # 7

"Boy, I tell you. I'm so goddamned mad. There it was, Saturday night and I get this pain in my belly, and I tried to get Dr. Jones. I've been going to him for years. I pay my bills on time and every other goddamned thing you're supposed to do right; and it took four hours to get the bastard, and then he was so unconcerned—sent some goddamned medicine out. I was up all night. I tell you, *doctors!*"

Stimulus # 8

"Every time I come home from a trip I think, well, that's the last time. I'm not going to cheat on Helen anymore. I'm really going to try to make a go of this marriage. I mean, I really want a relationship with her where there's just no room for anybody else, but by the time I'm home a week I realize what little we have in common. You know what I mean? Have you ever tried to interest your wife in one of your hobbies or tell her about your work and have her just change the subject? The way Helen goes around looking like the devil when this good-looking little gal comes along and is interested in everything you do and she fixes herself up because she knows she's going to see you. It makes you feel great. What would you personally do? You, you must have opportunities like that. Do you take advantage of them?

Stimulus # 9

"I'm tired of trying to work things out, really. It seems hopeless. I mean if there were a solution, that would be one thing, but there isn't. If I go back to him I could never really be the wife he wants. Nobody could be. He has these impossible ideas. Do you know what he's doing right now? Everyday he drinks himself into oblivion. He says without me he doesn't care what happens, and he makes me feel so responsible for his condition. Oh, God, I wish I could take enough of those pills that I'd die."

Stimulus # 10

"You know, last night I was thinking how much progress I've made. It all began six months ago. The time I was looking at my coffee pot, and for the first time I really saw it. And you know how it is now, how I hear the birds sing and I look at people and they're really there as people, and best of all, I'm really there. I'm not only there, but right now I'm here. You know the other day I was standing in the art gallery looking at a picture and a man came up and said, 'Gauguin is very nice, isn't he?' and so I said, 'I like you too.' "

The students' responses are spliced on an audiotape in a way that allows the class to listen to a stimulus statement and then all the responses before going on to the next stimulus statement. Here, again, the participants discuss each response in a critical way. Some of these statements raise difficult issues such as intense demands for direct help (Stimulus # 3) or overt seductiveness (Stimulus # 5). Many of the students sound strange or artificial in their taped responses, and there is a lot of anxiety. Often, they identify correctly the content and affect, but their own vocal qualities are stilted or wooden.

It might be helpful to appreciate the variability of the responses to look at representative responses to one of these stimuli statements. Stimulus # 7 is, on the surface, concerned with overt anger at doctors. At the minimum, one expects the beginning students to hear and reflect this aspect of the patient's communication. At least two other issues, however, are raised by the stimulus. The first involves the possibility that, at a different level, the patient is struggling with some type of fear about the pain in his abdomen. The second involves the possibility that the anger towards Doctor Jones and doctors in general may reflect anger toward the therapist. Both of these possibilities involve inference, and students are encouraged at this early stage of training to be aware of such possibilities without leaping to conclusions. Their responses might invite exploration of these possibilities, although focusing primarily on the overt affect and content. Representative responses might include the following:

> *Student # 1*: You were hurting and needed your doctor and when he wasn't available it made you very angry at him.
> *Student # 2*: Well, doctors are human and you shouldn't be too critical.
> *Student # 3*: He really didn't seem concerned—I wonder if it wasn't kind of scary . . . and . . . then the anger . . .
> *Student # 4*: Angry—angry as hell at him—doctors in general—can you feel some of it right now with me . . .?

The response from the first student is considered a reasonable one that meets the minimum requirements of the exercise. The second student made a destructive, non-empathic and guilt-inducing response. The third student "reached" for the presumed fear, and the fourth student's response invited the patient to explore the here-and-now aspects of the patient's communication. These four responses represent the range of responses to the second set of stimuli statements seen during each year's seminar.

Following this exercise, a third series of statements is presented. These, however, are videotaped rather than audiotaped. Volunteer nursing students, secretarial staff, and professionals are presented as patients, and each presents a stimulus to which the participants respond. Once again, the responses are audiotaped, and the tapes are played for group discussion. This exercise intro-

duces the complex area of nonverbal communication. One videotape, for example, presents an obviously pained and desperate
woman who can't seem to speak. Another presents an angry young
man. A third presents a young woman who states that she is angry
about sexual discrimination in the office, but smiles throughout
her statement. The students are thereby introduced to the concept
of conflicting messages and the technique of confrontation.* The
eight videotaped stimuli increase the students' appreciation of the
complexities of communication and give them an opportunity to
form specific responses in various real-life situations.

The major task of the student in these first three exericses is to
learn cognitive empathy. By the end of the third exercise, most of
the participants have become much more sensitive to manifest or
surface affect and have begun to feel more comfortable making
reflective statements. Each of the exercises, however, is a series
of two-statement exchanges: stimulus and response. In order to
introduce the group to some sense of longer interchanges, they
next view two videotaped exploratory interviews of a real patient
by two different psychiatrists. One psychiatrist does a collaborative, affect-focused type of interview, and the other a directive,
history-taking interview. The patient, a young, depressed woman
with a few verbal skills, was not known to either psychiatrist.
The class sees that it is possible to sustain a more reflective, affect-
centered interview, and that the different interviewing approaches
obtain useful—although different—types of data. They also note
that different types of relationships appear to evolve as the result
of the interviewing style of each psychiatrist. There was a suggestion, for example, that the directive psychiatrist came to feel
increasing responsibility for the patient. The instructor needs to
emphasize the usefulness of both styles, but stress that they have
different goals. The style tends to establish the type of therapist-
patient relationship.

The group also watches an affect-focused interview by Carl
Rogers, and contrasts it with a much more content-oriented and
interpretive psychoanalytic interview. Striking differences are

---

* See Chapter 7 for a discussion of training in confrontation.

noted, and it is useful to stop the videotape from time to time during each interview and encourage the students to discuss what they are seeing.

The next phase of instruction involves the students in role play-ing. One student plays the interviewer and the other plays the patient. No instructions are given to the "patient." The inter-viewer attempts to conduct a ten-minute, affect-focused, colla-borative interview. The students learn that, despite a concern with affect and cognitive empathy, there are many occasions in the interview in which the therapist must decide which of multiple messages to attend. They are able to see that at such decision points (or "Y's" in the road), they are inclined to encourage the patient (albeit subtly) to take a direction which is more familiar and comfortable for the therapist.

By this time in the exercises, it is becoming apparent to the students that the role of therapist requires multiple levels of atten-tion. Listening for affect is but one; the therapist also needs to follow the train of the patient's thoughts; note major themes within the interview, recognize obvious defenses, and become sen-sitive to nonverbal cues. Students often articulate amazement at the complexity of a two-person interaction and excitement about this learning.

In many ways, the next exercise provokes the most anxiety. An actor or actress is employed for several days, and each student does a 30-minute exploratory interview which is videotaped. The actor is instructed to imagine that a love affair has recently ter-minated and that he or she has been feeling sad, has not been sleeping well, and has lost interest in work. In every other way, the actor is encouraged to be spontaneous and to follow wherever the interview seems to go. The students are told that they will each interview the same patient and will be able to note the various ways in which they individually influence the course of an interview. (If they ask about the patient they are told he or she is an actor; if they do not ask, the information is not given.)

Four or five interviews are scheduled on successive days and, when all are completed, the students, as a group, view each and critique it. The interviews themselves are, of course, very different in quality. Although most are adequate, a few are either very good or very bad. One young male first-year resident, for example, was interviewing an aggressively seductive young female actress. She used her body in a way that was openly erotic; he, in turn, became increasingly tense, showed a marked increase in his own motor activity and, midway through the interview, switched to a very directive question-and-answer format. In the discussion following, he shared with the group how very anxious the "patient" made him, how he began to experience sexual fantasies about her, and how he was not aware during the interview that he had switched to the directive style in order to maintain control over both the interview and his anxiety-producing sexual fantasies.

Another example involved a young female student who was interviewing a young male actor. The interview went well, and it became apparent to all that he explored increasingly what appeared to be his own real feelings associated with an earlier loss. After the interview, the "patient" said, "This interview was different than the others. Somehow with this doctor I found myself forgetting your instructions, and talking about my real experiences of some years ago. I felt involved at a different level—I wasn't acting."

The participants are impressed with how much the interviewer influences the nature and outcome of the interview. They also have the opportunity to see themselves on videotape. This may lead to a variety of insights. One young woman, for example, could see the stiffness of her posture. Although she had received this comment from the group during the role-playing exercises, by seeing herself she could begin to appreciate better the impact of this postural message upon her interaction with the patient. Another example involved a young man participant who, when faced with the openly erotic movements of the actress, began to play with the zipper on his boot. He was not aware of this behavior until he saw it on the videotape replay of the interview.

I would not want to understate the pain involved in this type of learning. This increases the need for the instructor to provide a model of criticism without attack. The group itself (partly, I believe, because of the self-disclosure and pain) becomes a meaningful group for most of the participants. Often, in retrospect, they comment on the uniqueness of a group experience in which they receive a great deal of criticism, but rarely, if ever, feel personally attacked. The degree of group cohesiveness and mutual support varies for each year's group, but most often it is an important aspect of the seminar.

There are two additional exercises. One involves a forced fantasy procedure, and the other is the use of Kagan's (22) Interpersonal Process Recall Procedure. Although both of these have direct implications for understanding the feelings of the therapist and, therefore, affective empathy, they will be described in Chapter 6 which deals with awareness of the process of the therapist-patient interaction. Following these two procedures, the experiential part of the seminar switches to interviews with actual patients who are in a hospital. These interviews are conducted behind a one-way mirror, and each student does three to five of them. The patients who participate do so voluntarily and are told that the interview is part of a training seminar and that others will observe behind the mirror.

Each student monitors a particular aspect of the interview and reports his observations to the group at the conclusion of the interview. One may focus on the therapist's level of empathy, others on major themes, mechanisms of defense, nonverbal behavior, or other aspects of the interaction. By this time, the focus of the seminar has broadened to include a dozen or so variables derived from the four schools of psychiatry. These will be described in subsequent chapters.

At this point in the seminar, the participants have incorporated the construct of cognitive empathy. They are sensitive to the feelings of the patient and skillfully reflect the feelings in ways that facilitate the patient's increasing exploration. The task of the teacher now is to move the participants in the direction of affective empathy. This involves encouraging them to feel "with" patients at certain moments during the interview. As noted earlier, this capacity to "let go" is not achieved easily. One approach that I have used is to ask one of the observing residents to formulate a fantasy about the patient being interviewed by a colleague. At the conclusion of the interview, he or she shares this with the group. Most often, others add fantasy material of their own or comment on shared or idiosyncratic feelings about the patient. The instructor does the same thing, and increasingly it becomes legitimate to have feelings and fantasies about patients.

The level of affective arousal which is a part of affective empathy is, however, frequently anxiety-provoking for the beginning therapist. This is illustrated in the following vignette from a supervisory session of a second-year resident (23).

> A second-year resident in the 40th hour of twice-weekly therapy with a young woman reintegrating from a psychotic episode had consistently offered high levels of cognitive empathy. In a supervisory session a current recording revealed a marked decline in his empathic communications. The discussion which ensued revealed the resident's growing "boredom" with the patient's obsessively tinged material regarding her lack of casual, social skills. He acknowledged a sense of irritation and wondered if it was related to his own feelings of mild discomfort in certain social settings. He indicated that he was particularly surprised at his low-level empathic responses because in the preceding hour, for the first time, he had really experienced strong feelings with the patient. During that hour she had been describing intense loneliness, and he found himself remembering and feeling his own earlier intense loneliness. It became apparent to both of us that this different, deeper level of empathy had, for a number of reasons, frightened him and led to a retreat characterized by boredom, mild irritation, and failure to respond with even cognitive empathy to her communications.

As the seminar enters its final phases, most of the participants become more comfortable doing interviews behind a one-way mirror and begin to note spontaneously those moments during the interview when their own feelings were strong. "His anger made me anxious, but when we got to his sadness I felt really with him. I felt sad and briefly remembered a tough period earlier in my life. He really didn't want to explore his sadness though—did you notice how quickly he was back into his anger?" This type of self-report is not unusual during the latter stages of the seminar.

There are a number of reading assignments and group discussions of that literature despite the fact that most of the time is spent in exercises of different specific skills—in "doing." The articles reviewed assist in giving the participants a cognitive structure with which to understand that which they are doing. As noted earlier, Eisenberg's article (24) on the human nature of human nature is the initial reading and serves as a stimulus for a group discussion of the impact of the therapist's values upon the process of psychotherapy. Following this, the group reads a series of articles about empathy. We start with Carkhuff's (9) writings about cognitive empathy. They are clear and concrete. After this, the students read several psychoanalytic writers, in particular, Greenson (3) and Schafer (4). Havens' paper (2) on the existential use of the self introduces the group to the existential school of psychiatry and its position on empathy. Katz's chapter (21) on the effective empathizer is read also. This brief sampling of the literature on empathy gives the students a representative range of writing about this subject.

To recapitulate, the seminar starts with a single focus on learning empathy and, after several months, broadens to include other therapeutic processes and techniques. The group starts with a series of learning experiences and reading assignments about cognitive empathy. Within several months, they are more tuned to affective signals from the patient and come to realize that each participant has difficulties with various specific affects or content areas. One may deal effectively with anger, but not with helplessness, another may be able to deal with sadness, but not with anger. Another may respond sensitively to statements having to do with sexuality, but consistently avoid the issue of aging. This person-specific knowledge is of great importance to each individual. It points the way to blind spots, and if they do not give way to the impact of the educational experience, the resident may decide to enter personal psychotherapy or psychoanalysis. Self-awareness, in general, increases, and the group offers helpful feedback to each individual regarding his or her style of relating both to patients and within the group. Despite this aspect of the seminar, it is not group psychotherapy. There is considerable structure and a major commitment to an educational format.

All the processes, skills, or techniques seem unnatural to the students initially. They tend to feel artificial or even phoney. Some articulate anger at the instructor—"I don't feel like myself—I'm only doing this to please you, and that makes me mad." I respond by indicating that I expect they will put the skills together in their own ways. The skills, however, are necessary if they are to do effective psychotherapy and, like anything newly learned, will seem awkward and artificial at first. I insist that they will feel more natural later, and that does evolve for most students. The skills become their own, and many go on to experience affective empathy with their patients. I believe these young professionals are the therapists for the deeply regressed patients of tomorrow. Those who have difficulty in being deeply with their patients (or, for that matter, their own affect) would do better to seek other pursuits that do not require the ability to deal with deep and often frightening feelings.

During the latter stages of the seminar, each participant is assigned as psychotherapist to three patients. He or she also meets weekly with three different supervisors, and the second important experience of learning psychotherapy begins. Supervision and the lessons learned in the seminar are seen as complementary. The students take tape recordings and a written summary of each patient session to their supervisory meeting. Each supervisor's particular focus (countertransference, interpretive work, etc.) augments the beginning therapist's growing skills.

During the early stages of the seminar, there is little emphasis on psychodynamics. Rather, the stress is on manifest feelings and content, observational skills, and the stimulus impact of the therapist in evoking certain material. In this emphasis, the seminar follows the lead of Schlessinger, Muslin, and Baittle (25) who teach observational skills in a similar way. Later in the seminar, a psychodynamic focus is added, and one resident, for example, is asked to do a dynamic formulation following the observation of a colleague's interview.

It appears clear to the writer that empathy can be learned.

Initially, students have different levels of freedom and discipline with feelings and, as one might anticipate, those who enter psychotherapy training with greater native propensity appear to learn the most. All, however, appear to learn something about both psychotherapy and themselves.

REFERENCES

1. ISAACS, K. S., and HAGGARD, E. A., "Some Methods Used in the Study of Affect in Psychotherapy." In: L. A. Gottschalk and A. H. Auerbach (eds.), *Methods of Research in Psychotherapy*, 226-239. New York: Appleton-Century-Crofts, 1966.
2. HAVENS, L. L., "The Existential Use of the Self." *American Journal of Psychiatry*, 131:1, 1-10, January, 1974.
3. GREENSON, R. R., "Empathy and Its Vicissitudes." *International Journal of Psychoanalysis*, 41:418-424, 1960.
4. SCHAFER, R., "Generative Empathy in the Treatment Situation." *The Psychoanalytic Quarterly*, 28:3, 242-371, 1959.
5. PAUL, N. L., "The Use of Empathy in the Resolution of Grief." *Perspectives in Biology and Medicine*, Vol. 11, pp. 153-169, 1967-68.
6. LAUGHLIN, H. P., *The Neuroses*. Washington: Butterworth, 1967.
7. ROGERS, C. R., *On Becoming a Person*. Boston: Houghton Mifflin, 1961.
8. ROGERS, C. R., and TRUAX, C. B., "The Therapeutic Conditions Antecedent to Change: A Theoretical View." In: C. R. Rogers (ed.), *The Therapeutic Relationship and Its Impact*. Madison: University of Wisconsin Press, 1967.
9. CARKHUFF, R. R., *Helping and Human Relations*. Vol. I & II, New York: Holt, Rinehart & Winston, Inc., 1969.
10. BACHRACH, H. M., "Empathy: We Know What We Mean But What Do We Measure?" *Archives of General Psychiatry*, Vol. 33, 35-38, January, 1976.
11. ORLINSKY, D. E., and HOWARD, K. I., *Varieties of Psychotherapeutic Experience: Multivariate Analyses of Patients' and Therapists' Reports*. New York and London: Teachers College Press, Teachers College, Columbia University, 1975.
12. MUSLIN, H. L., "Clinical Exercises in Empathy." *Diseases of the Nervous System*, 35:8, 384-387, August, 1974.
13. CHARNY, E. J., "Psychosomatic Manifestations of Rapport in Psychotherapy." *Psychosomatic Medicine*, 28:4, Part I, July-August, 1966.
14. DiMASCIO, A., BOYD, R. W., and GREENBLATT, M., "Physiological Correlates of Tension and Antagonism During Psychotherapy." *Psychosomatic Medicine*, 19:99-104, 1957.
15. STRUPP, H. H., FOX, R. E., and LESSER, K., *Patients View Their Psychotherapy*. Baltimore: Johns Hopkins University Press, 1969.
16. CHESSICK, R. D., *How Psychotherapy Heals*. New York: Science House, 1969.
17. CHESSICK, R. D., *Why Psychotherapists Fail*. New York: Science House, 1971.

18. HALPERN, H. M., and LESSER, L. N., "Empathy in Infants, Adults, and Psychotherapists." *Psychoanalytic Review*, 47(3):32-42, 1960.
19. HENRY, W. E., SIMS, J. H., and SARAY, S. L., *The Fifth Profession.* San Francisco: Jossey-Bass, 1971.
20. MUSLIN, H. L., and SCHLESSINGER, N., "Toward the Teaching and Learning of Empathy." *Bulletin of the Menninger Clinic*, 35(4), pp. 262-271, July, 1971.
21. KATZ, R. L., "The Effective Empathizer," 134-160. In: *Empathy, Its Nature and Uses.* The Free Press of Glencoe: Collier-Macmillan, Ltd., 1963.
22. KAGAN, N., *Studies in Human Interaction*, 3 Vols., U.S. Dept. H.E.W., (ED107946), December, 1967.
23. LEWIS, J. M., "Practicum in Attention to Affect: A Course for Beginning Psychotherapists." *Psychiatry*, 37:2, pp. 109-113, May, 1974.
24. EISENBERG, L., "The Human Nature of Human Nature." *Science*, 176:4031, pp. 123-128, April 14, 1972.
25. SCHLESSINGER, N., MUSLIN, H. L., and BAITTLE, M., "Teaching and Learning Psychiatric Observational Skills." *Archives of General Psychiatry*, 18, 549-552, May, 1968.

CHAPTER 3

++

Respect, Warmth,

and Genuineness

++

++++++++++++++++++++++++++++ ++H

The variables to be described in this chapter—respect, warmth, and genuineness—are seldom thought of as something that can be taught. More often, they are considered as relatively fixed personality characteristics, and there has been relatively little attention paid to them in any systematic way in psychotherapy training programs. There are many reasons for the inattention to these variables. The four major schools of psychotherapy take positions regarding them that are at variance with each other. Although all of the schools espouse respect for the patient, the issue of how warm and how genuine the therapist should be is debated vigorously.

The objective-descriptive school does not speak directly to this question, although the role model of the optimal therapist is the expert, and the patient is the recipient of a respectful examination and treatment. Under most circumstances, because interpersonal distance is great, genuineness does not present a problem, and the warmth of the therapist is often masked by a professional role.

The psychoanalytic school emphasizes clear respect for the patient. The therapist's neutrality and objectivity are dominant forces in the relationship, and many view warmth as something that may interfere with the evolution of transference. As a rule, this school does not encourage therapist spontaneity and sharing of thoughts and feelings, or other expressions of genuineness. More recently, the emphasis has shifted from the therapist as the recipient of transference projections to the dimensions of the therapeutic alliance, somewhat diluting the mandate for neutrality and objectivity.

The interpersonal school, with its emphasis on the therapist as an active expert, often suggests a manipulative aspect to the therapist's behavior. Havens (1) has commented that there is a manipulative element in the operations of all psychotherapies, and the interpersonalists are distinguished on this score only by candor. At any rate, there is little emphasis on therapist genuineness in this school. Actually, at times, it may be permissible for the interpersonal therapist to mock, scorn, or in other ways to act quite disrespectfully to the patient. This is said to be primarily disrespect for the patient's projections to the therapist rather than for the patient's person—a tenuous distinction at best. The therapist of the interpersonal school always strives to behave in a way that makes the patient's projections impossible, and this takes precedence over the therapist's being warm, respectful, and genuine.

The existential school represents the most extreme departure from objectivity, neutrality, and professionalism. The therapist, in the attempt to be and stay with the patient, struggles to cast aside all preconceptions or hypotheses about the patient, and to meet the patient where he is. This is thought to be highly respectful to the patient and to involve high levels of genuineness and warmth.

It is apparent that what one can know or infer about the stances of the four schools suggests considerable differences in the positions they take regarding warmth and genuineness and a more general agreement (perhaps excluding the interpersonal school) about the proper role of respect in the psychotherapeutic transaction. If we look at those factors which seem to influence the level of the beginning therapist's respect, warmth, and genuineness, four factors stand out: the student's general level of psychological functioning; the degree to which the student has assumed a narrowly defined professional role; the system characteristics of the training program; and the specific attention to these variables in course work, seminars, or supervision.

Experience with resident psychiatrists and graduate students suggests that the general level of psychological functioning of individual students varies in important ways. Students functioning below a certain general level of personality integration cannot, as the result of an educational experience, alter the way they relate to others, having little freedom with which to experiment with little-used aspects of their own personalities. Determining this level in a given individual is difficult, and even training programs with high ratios of applicants to positions may occasionally accept an individual whose functioning does not permit the freedom for this very special type of learning. Often, these are very bright, highly intellectual, and somewhat rigid individuals whose difficulties with their own feelings preclude their being effective intensive psychotherapists. Conversely, one occasionally sees beginning students who have unusual access to their own feelings but manifest great difficulty in being objective or analytic. Errors in the selection of candidates for training are often due to a failure to discern their excessive rigidity or inadequate internal control.

In addition to the student's general level of psychological maturity, the impact of the internalization of a professional role that is too narrowly defined is a significant factor in his or her subsequent development. Most reasonably mature beginning residents, for example, have to some degree begun to experience themselves as professionals after the model of medical school. This partially incorporated role model has much value, but for some has crystalized an attitude toward the patient as an object or as the carrier of a disease. A diagnostic "mind-set" of great inter-

personal distance may have evolved which demonstrates respect
for the patient's disease rather than for the patient as person. For
reasonably mature residents, this set does not preclude the development of greater freedom to be warm and genuine, but it is difficult to overcome.

Impressionistically, there is an inverse correlation between the
student's level of psychological maturity and the degree to which
he or she clings to this previously incorporated, but no longer
useful, role model. Although individual exceptions are noted, it is
hard to escape the conclusion that education produces change
effectively only at certain levels of maturity. For students who
are less fortunate, personal therapy, with its increased emotional
arousal and opportunities for learning, may provide the best
possible solution.

Another factor which influences the levels of respect, warmth,
and genuineness in trainees concerns system characteristics of the
training program. This context which the student enters either
encourages the student's personal growth or reinforces the incorporation of a rigid professional role model. In this way, the social
system presents the beginning resident with messages about a
pattern of preferred, system-syntonic qualities. Some training
programs encourage warmth and genuineness, while others emphasize a more distant professional role model. The pattern of
social system characteristics in itself may be clear, or ambiguous,
or conflicting. The student is more comfortable when the system
characteristics are clear and, unless they prescribe an overly narrow definition of the "way to be," this circumstance is conducive
to growth. Ambiguous or conflicting system messages about a preferred or ideal type often lead to considerable confusion and
anxiety on the part of the students.

Relatively few training programs address themselves specifically to the variables of respect, warmth, and genuineness. One
exception is the description of training exercises by Rogers, Truax,
and Carkhuff (2, 3, 4). These three variables are important aspects of psychotherapeutic functioning, and training programs
benefit their students by being explicit in regard to both the range

of possible role models and the preferred, or ideal, model in their particular setting.

RESPECT

In this seminar, there is considerable emphasis placed upon the trainees' learning what kinds of behavior communicate respect or, conversely, some degree of disrespect to their psychotherapy patients. Respecting another person has many meanings. One common usage implies a debt, perhaps for some special talent or status. There may be an almost begrudging quality in that definition of respect. As the term is used in this seminar, however, it has more to do with individual boundaries—that is, the patient's way of feeling, thinking, and responding. It does not imply agreement with that which the individual feels or thinks but, rather, a regard for the right of the other person to act in accord with personal perceptions, both from within and without. The therapist may find himself or herself in disagreement with the patient's perceptions and conclusions. At such times, the therapist may choose to acknowledge that disagreement. If this leads to an exploration of various ways to interpret particular events, it will offer an opportunity for therapist and patient to negotiate a shared meaning. Negotiation is a very respectful process in which there is no attempt to overpower the patient's perception or force the therapist's conclusion upon him. In this way, respect involves sharing power, and it facilitates a basic collaboration between therapist and patient. Unless the therapist respects the right of the patient to see things the patient's way, there is no basis for consensual validation or for the patient to experience individual boundaries (both his own and others').

If the therapist feels that, by virtue of professional training, an expertise has developed that carries with it a private claim to "the truth"; if the therapist's view of reality is inevitably the "right" view; if he or she presumes to know the patient's thoughts, feelings, or meaning with absolute certainty, the therapist not only appears overpowering, but incapable of respect for views that differ from his or her own. If, on the other hand, "reality" is treated as a subjective affair, and differences are negotiated, the therapist will not only learn more about the patient, but will also demonstrate respect for the patient's ego boundaries and an appreciation of how the patient experiences the world.

Another aspect of respect is that it communicates a consideration of the patient's potential for future mastery. "At this time you feel overwhelmed with your loss," or "Right now, it seems impossible" are statements that focus on the temporal aspect of the patient's dilemma and imply that the patient can be and can feel differently in the future. Although subtle, the therapist's respect for the patient's potential can be powerfully therapeutic.

These two issues—the patient's right to perceive, feel, think, and respond in his or her own way, and the clear message that the patient has the potential for change—are the basic ways in which the seminar addresses the development of respect in beginning psychotherapists. There are no specific exercises aimed at the development of respect, but from the beginning of the seminar and with the exercises aimed at the learning of cognitive empathy, the instructor introduces the concept of respect. Respect for the patient's boundaries and potential is most conspicuous when it is absent. The student who appears inattentive, preoccupied, or bored is confronted with these observations. Even during the early tape-recorded responses to single patient statements, the quality of the student's voice can reveal his or her regard. Carkhuff (4) has pointed out that respect is communicated in the degree of attention and the tonal qualities of the therapist's responses rather than directly in words. The students in the seminar rapidly develop the ability to confront each other with their observations about the level of respect. Often, the group learns through discussion of such observations that what appears on the surface to be (and is) lack of respect on the part of the beginning therapist is often experienced by that therapist as anxiety.

Another area in which the presence or absence of respect is clearly demonstrated is in the therapist's interpretations.* It is when the focus is on the meaning of the patient's behavior that one is most apt to see the unskilled and disrespectful use of

* See Chapter 7 for a discussion of interpretation.

power by the beginning therapist. However, in films even experienced and well-known therapists may come across as powerful, invasive, and either uninterested in the patient's understanding of his behavior or unimpressed with anything but their own insights. These therapists seem so certain and so powerful that there appears to be little need for further input from the patient: "Perhaps, but the real issue is your inability to be direct." "Alright, but we know that in this situation your anxiety always gets worse." "This is interesting, but I don't think it's important in this instance." Each of these examples contains an element of therapist's disrespect, implying that the therapist's understanding is far superior to the patient's.

Along with films of therapists whose interpretative work is like that described, the beginning students also have the opportunity to watch films of therapists who involve the patient collaboratively in a search for meaning. "I see the way it looks to you. Are there other possible meanings that come to your mind?" "I've wondered whether you've considered this possibility?" "It kind of looks this way to me—can we look at it from both perspectives?"

Viewing films of psychotherapy interviews becomes of increasing value to the students as they begin to learn what variables to attend. Actually, until specific variables are introduced in the seminar, students tend to watch films of psychotherapy interviews without knowing exactly what to look for. They quickly become sensitive to a therapist's respect for the patient's boundaries and potential in films that demonstrate wide variations in this variable; then they become sensitive to their own, as well as others', communications with patients.

Consideration of respect for the patient brings up those therapists who appear to act deliberately in ways that are patently disrespectful to the patient. Havens (1) discusses this in relationship to Sullivan's counterprojective techniques. In these attempts to distinguish what the patient projects to the therapist and to deal directly with such transferred material by acting against it, the interpersonal therapist may often be disrespectful in manner. According to Havens, Sullivan was "mocking, sarcastic, and off-hand . . ." Watching the films of an interpersonal therapist and his counterprojective maneuvers during a psychotherapy interview may lead students to feel that there are many moments of patent disrespect.

For beginners, the seminar must emphasize the importance of communicating respect rather than licensing disrespect, even if considered a counterprojective technique. Becoming an interpersonal therapist may be thought of as an advanced goal or skill, but for the beginning therapist counterprojective maneuvers appear to provide some type of rationale for what may well be the angry or rejecting feelings of the therapist towards the patient. For that reason, it appears unwise to encourage a technique for beginners that has great potential for misuse.

WARMTH

One of the more controversial aspects of the process of psychotherapy is whether or not to communicate warmth or caring directly. Few would argue with the idea that the therapist should be interested, even concerned; but how much warmth should he or she feel and communicate? Part of this problem results from the differing concepts of warmth in a relationship. Under most circumstances, warmth is a quality of emotional intensity that signals that one likes or cares about another. Strupp (5) has constructed a useful five-point bipolar scale of the therapeutic climate. At the midpoint is neutrality in which the therapist's attitude is objective and task-oriented. At one end of the scale is warmth, and at this point the therapist's attitude is one of acceptance, understanding, and tolerance. If the therapist's attitude is usually warm, the patient comes to feel highly regarded. The message of warmth in this instance is, "I like you." Beavers (6) has suggested, however, that need is communicated also. The message is not only, "I like you," but also, "I, too, have a need to be liked." In these terms, warmth is both positive regard for another and an invitation for him to reciprocate. It is precisely this expression of the therapist's need that appears to precipitate the controversy. Some writers see the patient's needs as the fundamental basis for the psychotherapeutic process and consider any intrusion of the therapist's needs to have potentially destructive implications. This may be an impossible demand upon the therapist, and may have played a role in the development of the concept of absolute neutrality. If taken to an extreme, such neutrality denies humanness. Of course, there are limits to the extent to which it is appropriate for the therapist's needs to be involved. I referred earlier to the therapist whose personal life is so bereft of gratification that he or she turns increasingly to patients to satisfy personal needs. I would reemphasize the importance of the therapist's intimate, interpersonal, social network, for without such support the therapist may experience a strong pull to use patients as a source to fulfill these needs. This possibility of misuse, however, should not blind us to the type of general fulfillment that occurs appropriately in relationships with patients.

Kagan's (7) work with the interpersonal process recall technique has suggested that both patient and therapist are often concerned with how they are being regarded. These concerns are said to be inevitable in any relationship. The mandate to the therapist is not to deny the presence and gratification of his or her needs, but to be fully aware of their impact upon the relationship, their potential for misuse, and the ways in which they may interfere with the primary goals of therapy.

Most beginning residents have considerable warmth which often has not been encouraged in the course of earlier education. For these, a training program that encourages this type of openness enables them to experience this aspect of psychotherapy training as a renewed freedom to be more naturally themselves. Those few who are not naturally warm usually follow one of two patterns. The more common type is the resident whose own needs are so intense and threatening that he must relate with excessive impersonality and great distance. The second type is the resident who relates with overwhelming intensity and whose underlying hunger impedes the psychotherapeutic transaction.

In summary, warmth, defined to include both positive regard for another and the communication of a personal need, is not something that one either has or has not. With few exceptions, beginning therapists need only to be put in touch with this aspect of themselves; its expression needs to be legitimized. For a few, being in touch with and communicating either positive regard or their own needfulness are threatening. Whether they present themselves as cold and remote or excessively loving, change is necessary if they are to become therapists. Often, intensive psychotherapy or psychoanalysis with its potential for personality change is the fruitful approach.

A rule of thumb might suggest that unless a therapist sees something about the patient that is likeable or comes to feel an increasing sense of caring during early interviews, the patient should be referred to another therapist. This coming to value the patient is implemented by the empathic process—that is, the ability to place oneself in another's situation. To feel with another brings the therapist an increasing understanding of the patient and his dilemma. With such understanding comes the potential for caring and ultimately warmth. It is frequently a surprise to beginning therapists to note the development of warmth in regard to certain patients. One first-year resident said it well, "I would not have believed I could ever feel this way about this woman." He was referring to a very obese, middle-aged, angry, dependent, alcoholic woman with whom initial psychotherapy hours had evoked anxiety, distance, and moderate disgust.

There are no specific exercises for the development of warmth but, as with respect, during the earlier segments of the seminar the instructor introduces the construct in his critique of the students' responses to the exercise. One rarely finds an appropriate opportunity to directly inform another that one cares about him or her. Rather, warmth is more often noted in its absence and, in particular, in the remote and presumably objective professional model. The therapist who responds to the patient's affective message with "under certain circumstances you appear to feel rather lonely" is less apt to communicate warmth than the therapist who states, "It sounds terribly lonely." So much, however, of the therapist's warmth is communicated in ways other than with words that it is difficult to convey it in written form. "Drop dead," for example, can be said in a warm and caring way just as "I like

you" can communicate anger or disgust. The tremendous importance of the ways in which each of us qualifies or negates verbal
communication becomes increasingly obvious to the students as
the issue of the therapist's warmth is discussed.

A striking example of this type of disqualification occurred in
the tape-recorded response of one student to an early stimulus
statement. The student identified the affect and content of the
patient's message (elation regarding finding new friends), but in
reflecting it in the response, "You really sound happy about your
new friends," sounded wooden and remote. "Sam," one of the other
students said, "you sound like you're describing the microscopic
findings in hepatic cirrhosis."

GENUINENESS

Earlier, the problems presented by the incorporation of a narrowly defined role model were referred to. This model emphasizes
the emotional detachment of the beginning therapist from the patient. It is a necessary part of the professional's attitude about a
patient, and it is also, I believe, a necessary part of the psychotherapist's way of relating to the patient. With the emotional distance that it provides, it allows the therapist to appraise the patient's current functioning, psychodynamics, movement in therapy, as well as the quality of the therapist-patient interaction. It
is the essential counterbalance to the empathic process. The difficulty, however, is that the empathic process is not emphasized
in earlier educational experiences nor, for that matter, in any
systematic way in most psychotherapy training programs. As a
consequence, detachment may become the only way in which the
student learns to relate to a patient. Of course, the process is
more complicated than it appears because the use of the narrowly
defined, distant, detached role model can serve as a defense
against the closeness that is so much a part of the empathic
process. This incorporation of the role model into what is really
a neurotic process poses particular problems in the training of
psychotherapists.

The larger problem, however, is the tendency of many beginning therapists to convert the realistic need for recurring moments of detachment during each psychotherapy interview to a pervasive style of relating to the patient in a detached way. This can appear as excessively formal and has the potential for powerful impact on the patient-therapist interaction. It may invite the patient to relate to the therapist in a comparable way and reduce the likelihood of deeply shared, empathic moments. To further complicate the matter, the patient's responses to such cues may be labeled by the therapist as pathological, rather than as understandable responses to the therapist's signals.

The question of the therapist's spontaneity is vigorously debated. Although few teachers of psychotherapy encourage a consistently detached manner of relating, the objective-descriptive, psychoanalytic, and interpersonal schools emphasize detached skills or characteristics of the therapist. Indeed, if neutrality, for example, is carried to an extreme in the face of considerable patient discomfort, it can be seen as a device by which the therapist hides his or her own feelings. It may present the patient with conflicting messages from the therapist as, for example, when the therapist's neutrality is contradicted by subtle verbal or nonverbal cues that suggest other attitudes. Perhaps more than in any other psychotherapeutic system, psychoanalysis suggests that by not reacting (or grossly under-reacting) to what the patient says, the therapist is encouraging the development of transference. The position of this seminar is that transference is ubiquitous and should not be encouraged. Neutrality designed to encourage the development of a transference neurosis is a particular technique specific to formal psychoanalytic treatment and is ill suited to most psychotherapy. Encouraging this heightened degree of focus on the past upon the therapist may be essential in some treatment situations—namely, with individuals with many mature ego functions (such as psychoanalytic candidates) or perhaps in some severely disturbed and regressed individuals with psychoses or severe psychosomatic syndromes. In the latter instances, the transference may actually be more psychotic than neurotic, and there must be a commitment to many years of analytic work. A therapist should not undertake such a course—the deliberate invitation to such intense transference—without both the requisite psychoanalytic skills and the commitment to many years of work with the patient. For patient with moderate psychopathology, transference can be discouraged by the therapist's open presentation of himself or herself as a responsive, mistake-prone human who has certain understandings and skills to offer in a collaborative relationship. This does not mean, of course, that responding in such a fashion will prevent the emergence of the ubiquitous transference phenomenon, but it may diminish the likelihood of the development of severe transference fixations.

Those who take a strong position against therapist's genuineness may feel it implies an invitation to complete self-disclosure. This is not the intent; rather, what is encouraged is that the therapist be willing to react openly and honestly with his patient whenever there are no clear contraindications to such behavior. This leads to a general style of relating to patients which has, at its base, a high level of genuineness. Contraindications may relate to several issues. The first is when a therapist's spontaneous response appears to be harmful to the patient. The second involves a response of the therapist that has much more to do with the therapist's life situation outside of therapy than it does to the here-and-now interaction with the patient.

There is perhaps no aspect of psychotherapy training that gives beginning students more difficulty than being genuine. There is much more ease and safety in assuming the stereotyped professional role, and it is a natural position for most beginning students. In addition, students may have an image of the detached therapist seated quietly behind the patient on the couch. However distorted, this model may lure the beginning therapist into assuming a distant and objective attitude. With the exception of the existential approach, there is little to encourage genuineness. Even training programs that encourage therapists to be genuine in the encounter differ greatly on what the beginning therapist is taught to be genuine about. This, for the most part, involves the problem of self-disclosure* but is, I believe, a broader issue than self-

---

* See Chapter 4.

disclosure. The seminar asks the beginning therapists to be more genuinely themselves as professionals than the narrowly defined and distant role model. It suggests also that as they learn to be therapists they will feel more naturally and genuinely in their relationships with patients.

There are no specific exercises for genuineness and, once again, absence of genuineness, or what appears to be the assumption of a narrow and stereotyped professional role model, is what is often noted in the earlier segments of the training program. In the students' attempts, for example, to respond at certain levels of cognitive empathy to the manifest feelings of patients or to patient stimuli statements, one may note considerable contradiction. The student's words may express considerable sensitivity to what the patient is feeling, but the way in which the response is stated may suggest little real understanding. In addition to the instructor's comments about tone of voice, posture, etc., the other members of the group provide confrontation as well as support. As the seminar moves into the videotaped interviews with an actor and the interviews with actual patients, the students are able to comment very directly to one another about how genuine the student therapist seems to be: "You really seemed so different in that interview, Jeff, than you are either here in our group or as we have seen you in other interviews—you just didn't seem yourself." Gradually, this type of confrontation in regard to genuineness (as well as warmth and respect) brings to open discussion the quality of underlying anxiety that interferes with the encounter aspects of the interview. "The reason I seem so detached and unnatural is that I was anxious about some sexual feelings I was having about the patient." "I really was afraid of this patient—afraid that all his rage would explode right here in the interview." "I found myself trying to put great distance between us. He was so clinging and sucking, and the more anxious I felt about assuming responsibility for him, the more impersonal and distant I became." It is through the impact of the student's anxiety and associated fantasies that the other members of the group come to understand the nature of their own resistances to encounter. The more distinctive the patient's characteristics, the more likely that the students will share a common anxiety. The less distinctive the patient's impact, the greater the likelihood that there will be fewer shared (and more idiosyncratic) fantasies and anxieties.

As the students move into interviewing actual patients behind a one-way screen, the pervasive influence of each student's anxiety upon the the conduct of the interview becomes a central focus of the seminar. Openness within the group is encouraged, and the group, under most circumstances, provides a great deal of support. The clearest indicators of anxiety that interferes with the conduct of the interview occur when a student departs from his or her usual level of respect, warmth, and genuineness. At levels of greater anxiety, more obvious behavior appears. Nevertheless, the group's ability to perceive subtle variations in respect, warmth, and genuineness often helps the beginning therapist to be in touch with anxieties that have moved him or her back to a position of distance and stereotypical professionalism.

The seminar attempts to highlight the importance of a therapist's warmth, respect, and genuineness. He or she must be able to care about the patient as another human being and, in the process, must not be afraid of letting some personal human needs show. There must be respect for the patient's ego boundaries as reflected in his idiosyncratic feelings, thoughts, and fantasies, as well as a belief in his potential for change and growth. A therapist also must not be afraid to communicate genuine responses to that which transpires between therapist and patient. The clear feedback that this provides the patient is instrumental in helping the patient gain a sense of his or her impact upon at least one other human being. All of this is not to say, however, that the seminar licenses wild or irrational behavior on the part of the therapist. The explicit mandate is that the psychotherapeutic relationship with the patient is in the service of the patient's need for change and growth. The therapist must provide both the technical expertise to help the patient and the deeply human (and very intimate) relationship that makes the technical expertise helpful. Each without the other is of little use. It is useful to keep in mind the uniqueness of the psychotherapeutic venture. Strupp (5, p. 705) has said it well:

> At its best, individual psychotherapy creates conditions for such learning unequaled by anything human ingenuity has been able to devise, and it represents a powerful affirmation of the individual's worth, self-direction, and independence. While costly in terms of money, time, manpower, and dedication of the participants to the common task, it remains one of the few oases in a collectivistic society that fosters conformity and erodes individual values and autonomy in a host of ways. . . . In essence, it remains an unrealizable ideal of self-discovery through learning and teaching in the context of a human relationship uninfluenced by ulterior motives of indoctrination or social control.

REFERENCES

1. HAVENS, L. L., *Participant Observation*. New York: Jason Aronson, Inc., 1976.
2. ROGERS, C. R., *On Becoming a Person*. Boston: Hougton Mifflin, 1961.
3. TRUAX, C. B., and CARKHUFF, R. R., *Toward Effective Counseling and Psychotherapy: Training and Practice*. New York: Aldine, 1967.
4. CARKHUFF, R. R., *Helping and Human Relations*. Vol. I & II, New York: Holt, Rinehart & Winston, Inc., 1969.
5. STRUPP, H. H., *Psychotherapy: Clinical, Research, and Theoretical Issues*. New York: Jason Aronson, Inc., 1973.
6. BEAVERS, W. R., *Psychotherapy and Growth: A Family Systems Perspective*. New York: Brunner/Mazel, 1977.
7. KAGAN, N., *Studies in Human Interaction*, 3 Vols., U.S. Dept. H.E.W., (ED107946), December, 1967.

CHAPTER 4

+++

Self-Disclosure

+++

++

No aspect of psychotherapy provokes as much disagreement among therapists as self-disclosure. For that reason, in particular, beginning therapists need to be provided some orienting information and introduced to the complexity of the issue.

Some years ago there were no major disagreements. The need to orient beginners was less acute. Programs training psychiatrists taught therapists not to reveal themselves to patients in any way. The prevailing model of psychotherapy was psychoanalytic, and psychiatrists were taught never to share their feelings, attitudes, associations, or fantasies with a patient in order to remain neutral and allow transference to evolve in as uncomplicated a manner as possible. In the intervening years, there has been much ferment in the field of psychotherapy associated with the development of the "newer" therapies, some of which espouse rather complete openness on the part of the therapist. The broad range of degree of therapist's self-disclosure can be conceptualized as a continuum, which Weiner (1) describes as ranging from neutrality to nudity. In my judgment, including nudity and physical contact in the concept of self-disclosure confuses the issue. As discussed in this chapter, therapist's self-disclosure means the therapist's sharing with the patient his or her feelings, thoughts, associations, fantasies, or other personal mental content.

The issue of physical contact is a complicated one. For some, physical contact inevitably suggests sexuality, and a rigid "no touch" rule is seen as a way of avoiding this possibility. For others, however, there are forms of physical contact (a handshake, a pat on the shoulder) that have no erotic implication and may, under certain circumstances, be a part of psychotherapy. I recall attending a psychiatric meeting as a young psychiatrist at which the speaker addressed this issue. He stated that he routinely shook hands, patted patients' shoulders when he thought it helpful and, on rare occasions, hugged a patient at the end of their final session. The audience of psychiatrists applauded these statements.

The seminar students are told that there is no place in psychotherapy for any erotic or sexual contact. I suggest to them that the decision regarding non-sexual physical contact must be made on the basis of the assessment of the individual patient, the treatment alliance, transference and countertransference issues and, in general, the totality of the treatment situation. They are asked to consider, however, that either their inclination for non-sexual contact with all patients or a strong urge for such contact with particular patients suggests a strong possibility that they are dealing solely with their own needs.

The teacher of psychotherapy must introduce students to something more than guidelines about physical contact. Students should be introduced to the complexity of self-disclosure; and to do so an initial examination of the polar positions of two schools of psychotherapy represents a good introduction.

Psychoanalysis is identified most closely with the position of little, or no, self-disclosure. The emphasis on the therapist's neutrality in order not to complicate evolving transference is a central tenet of psychoanalysis. Disclosure is considered to demonstrate gratification of the transference, acting out countertransference, or a reflection of the therapist's narcissistic preoccupations. Implicit in these concerns is the concept that by reducing the analyst's activity, the danger of using patients to fulfill personal emotional needs is minimized. Namnum (2), a contemporary psychoanalytic writer, however, may reflect a change occurring within that field when he calls attention to the projection-inducing aspect of anonymity (pp. 111-112).

> So-called anonymity or incognito on the part of the analyst facilitates projections onto him, in the same way an unstructured field may induce the emergence of regressive mechanisms in the perception of external stimuli. This point relates, however, only to the perceptual, impersonal aspect of the process; it alone does not constitute a transference. A transference can only develop in the climate of a human, and to some degree reciprocal, relationship . . . The fact is that complete masking of the analyst's identity or absolute mirror-like neutrality or abstinence does not offer the best conditions for the analysis of transference phenomena.

Namnum states that the analyst's real image can serve as the background for the analysis of transference reactions. Although "certain facts of his private life" can remain anonymous, the analyst's "true nature" cannot really be kept secret from the patient. He then goes on to discuss the balance of involvement and distance central to the analytic task.

Greenson (3) has indicated that both spontaneity on the part of the analyst in responding to the patient's reality situation and clear acknowledgment of technical errors are acceptable forms of self-disclosure.

Despite, however, the evidence of increased attention to the therapeutic alliance and reciprocity within the relationship, the psychoanalytic school is still identified primarily by an extremely cautious position about self-disclosure. For the therapist to present himself or herself as a "real" person, spontaneously responding to sudden changes in the patient's real world, or acknowledging his or her errors is a long way from sharing deeply personal material with a patient.

It is no surprise to find existential psychiatry at the opposite pole. Evolving, in part, as a negative response to psychoanalytic neutrality, this basically subjective school encourages the therapist to share his private world (if it is in the service of being with the patient). Havens (4) has suggested that existential psychiatry offers the therapist the first systematic approach to self-disclosure. However, operationalizing this approach in a way that provides specific guidelines remains a problem. How, for example, does a therapist know if disclosure is in the service of being with the patient or in the service of gratifying his or her own needs?

These polar positions do not provide the beginner with much help unless he or she comes into training with a preformed commitment to a particular school of psychiatry. This may be true for those with an earlier personal psychotherapy or psychoanalysis. For most, however, there is no such early commitment, and the polar positions of psychoanalysis and existential psychiatry offer little assistance.

Research studies, as pointed out by Weiner (1), offer little help to the beginning therapist. There is the suggestion that in research involving nonpatients (5) high levels of self-disclosingness by the therapist are positively correlated with high levels of self-disclosingness by the research subjects. The relationships, if any, of such findings to psychotherapy and, in particular, to the outcome of psychotherapy are unclear. There are conflicting reports in the group psychotherapy literature (6, 7, 8) regarding the role of therapist's self-disclosure. Truax and Carkhuff (9) report that high levels of therapist's transparency in individual therapy are associated with increased patient self-explorations and clinical improvement. Other investigators (6, 8) report results that contradict these findings. In summary, there is little consistent support either for or against the value of therapist's self-disclosure in the research literature.

A confusion of terms further complicates understanding. Therapist's genuineness, for example, is often used interchangeably with self-disclosure. It is obvious, however, that a therapist may be genuinely himself or herself without disclosing personal feelings or fantasies. He or she may be natural, feel very genuine, react with considerable spontaneity, and yet not reveal directly private thoughts.

It appears that in order to be helpful to our students, rather than ask, "Should the therapist reveal himself or herself?" we need to ask, "Under what situations, with what patients might the therapist disclose what about himself or herself?" The answers to these questions would deal more precisely with the variables involved in such a consideration. These would include the nature of the treatment goals, the patient's level of psychopathology, the nature of the therapeutic relationship, the nature of the disclosure, and the context in which the disclosure may occur.

TREATMENT GOALS

Weiner (10) has divided psychotherapy into three types: repressive, ego-supportive, and evocative, implicitly suggesting that self-disclosure is most useful in ego-supportive therapy. The basic mechanism of this type of therapy is feedback, the therapist's communication to the patient of the therapist's reactions to him or her. Patients are encouraged to take responsibility for their own feelings (rather than to explore their evolution through understanding their transference to the therapist). In this way, ego-supportive therapy focuses primarily on the patient's interpersonal impact. In contrast, evocative therapy, with its emphasis on interpretation, involves greater deprivation (and consequently increased neutrality) on the part of the therapist. There is less concern with providing the patient with feedback of an interpersonal nature. On the other hand, in repressive therapy the therapist is less concerned also with the provision of interpersonal feedback and relies instead on direct teaching, reassurance, and positive coping mechanisms. Within Weiner's framework, the goals of psychotherapy are included in the decision about self-disclosure, but do not stand alone. Many exceptions come to mind: the chronic schizophrenic patient in once-a-month therapy

whose helpful identification with the therapist appears to be facili-
tated by certain self-disclosures to the patient, or the severe character disorder in three-times-a-week evocative therapy whose
therapist shares personal reactions to loss at a time when the
patient has lost someone important. It is apparent that the goals
of therapy need to be considered in conjunction with other factors
in the decision regarding self-disclosure.

LEVEL OF PSYCHOPATHOLOGY

The level of the patient's psychopathology is another important factor in the therapist's decision to disclose, although there
are no clear guidelines on the basis of this factor alone. Weiner
(10) points out that patients with few ego strengths have both
the potential for misinterpreting a therapist's disclosure and a
great need for certainty in the form of reality confrontations. In
this sense, they stand an opportunity either to gain or to be
damaged by a therapist's disclosure. Well-integrated, neurotic-
level patients can tolerate more without damage, but need less
input about reality. Some therapists may share their own private
fantasies with a deeply regressed patient in an effort to help them
distinguish reality from fantasy, whereas other therapists feel
free to disclose their own associations only in instances such as
in response to neurotic patients' dreams in the effort to deal with
the patient's resistances to further associations. Each group might
well consider the disclosures of the other group to be counter-
productive, even dangerous.

Additionally, there is not a perfect correlation between the goals
of treatment and the patient's level of psychopathology. Some
therapists treat very disturbed and regressed patients intensively
with the goal of considerable personality reorganization, while
other therapists treat the patients with the same level of psychopathology in a more supportive manner. No simple, two-variable
system involving the goals of treatment and the level of psychopathology will give clear guidelines for self-disclosure to the therapist who does not occupy a polar position on the self-disclosure
continuum.

THERAPEUTIC RELATIONSHIP

In considering this factor, the therapist must examine both the nature of the working alliance and the current and anticipated nature of the transference-countertransference elements of the therapy. Weiner (10) has suggested that a therapist's self-disclosures are safest when the alliance is neither strongly positive nor strongly negative. When the alliance is either strongly positive or negative, there is a likelihood that self-disclosures, regardless of their content, will only intensify the previous state of the alliance.

Transference and countertransference factors must be considered in the decision to self-disclose. The therapist must ask himself in what ways these aspects of the therapy impinge upon his decision. In my experience as a therapist, however, transference and countertransference are most obvious in that reflective period following a spontaneous disclosure. Such disclosures do occur and when they do, I ask myself, "Why did I say that?" "What is going on that I haven't been aware of or acknowledged to myself?" Even when the self-disclosure is thoughtful and carefully planned, it may reflect a response to transference or countertransference, but that is less likely than when it occurs spontaneously.

Although the nature of the relationship may influence the decision of the therapist to disclose, by itself it provides little in the way of definite indications and contraindications.

NATURE OF THE DISCLOSURE

There are some aspects of the therapist's life that can be disclosed insofar as what patients can deduce from the therapist's appearance, dress, office decor, professional reputation, and other sources of semi-public information. There is, however, a hierarchy of more personal information that some therapists share with some patients under certain circumstances. This hierarchy would start with identifying data such as age, marital status, parenthood, and other personal but not private data. Even at this relatively superficial level, there are differences of opinion. I recall an informal conference in which two experienced psychoanalytically oriented therapists responded to the question of how they would respond to a patient who asked in the first interview, "Doctor, do you have any children?" One indicated that he would respond, "Why do you ask?" and refuse to provide the answer. The other indicated that he would say, "Yes, three . . . why do you ask?" The first therapist defended his position by indicating that he did not wish to interfere with early transference, while the second argued the need for both a "real" relationship and the inquiry into the meaning of the question. Although such disagreement may appear to be a large fuss about a small matter, the issue of therapist's self-disclosure stirs up vigorously defended positions. For the trainees watching the interchange, the discussion confused the complex issue even further.

At a more personal level, the therapist may choose to disclose attitudes, opinions, and value judgments. I have referred earlier to Halleck's concern that patients have a right to know from the outset something of the ideology of the therapist. However, this type of self-disclosure provokes an increasing number of therapists who disapprove and feel that if the patient requests the information, the therapist should respond only with an inquiry designed to clarify the patient's motives.

Another level of self-disclosure involves the therapist's sharing personal experiences. This type of disclosure is most often used in some therapists' psychotherapy with adolescents or young adults. Often, it is explained on the basis that severely disturbed young people often have little in the way of a consensual validation of their experiences. To know that one's therapist also was afraid when he went from junior high school to the larger senior high school is thought to provide the patient with useful information of this type.

At an increasingly personal level is the concept of the therapist's sharing his or her associations to patient material. Those who use this technique do so based on the rationale that it is one method of dealing with the patient's resistance to exploration. These therapists point out that with certain patients, when repeated interpretation of the patient's resistances to exploration fail, the therapist may consider sharing certain of his associations to the material.

Feelings are shared by some therapists as they relate to the here-and-now relationship. This is said to be providing certain patients with a type of feedback regarding their impact upon others. In my experience, therapists who adopt primarily an interpersonal stance in their psychotherapeutic work are most apt to provide this type of feedback in a fairly routine way. Existential therapists are often disclosing of their own feelings if it is in the service of "being with" the patient.

At a deeply personal level, some therapists share their fantasies with certain patients. Under some circumstances Searles (11), for example, discloses fantasy material to schizophrenic patients in an effort to help them distinguish between fantasy and reality.

This type of hierarchy of degree of privacy is my own, and others might arrange the levels differently. With therapists (like other folk), the more personal the information, the less likely they are to reveal it. Some therapists, however, reveal highly personal material in very selective instances with a clear rationale and definite goals in mind. It is apparent, however, that despite the general trend, the degree of privacy itself does not provide clear guidelines for self-disclosure.

CONTEXT

Another variable that may influence a therapist's decision to self-disclose is the circumstance of the moment. Assuming that the therapist has considered all of the factors noted above, there remains the particular context to be considered. First, there may be a difference between disclosing in response to a patient's inquiry and volunteering information. Some therapists rarely volunteer, but may respond to a patient's questions. A second special context involves an unusual event in the life of a patient, such as a sudden loss of a loved one. Here, some therapists would volunteer their condolences in a simple and direct way. Others, however, would not. A third special context involves a significant event in the life of the therapist (such as a serious illness or loss). Even in these unusual circumstances there are disagreements as to whether the therapist should volunteer the information about himself or herself.

Clearly, the confusion and conflict in the field of psychotherapy regarding self-disclosure are the result of the complexity of the issue. There can be no simple guidelines when there are so many different ideologies and processes included under the rubric of psychotherapy. Weiner (10), for example, states that there are only three absolute indications for self-disclosure: 1) to preserve the life of either the patient or the therapist; 2) in situations where external events in the therapist's life have significantly influenced his feelings and the therapeutic relationship; and 3) a disruption in therapy due to some aspect of the therapist's personality or conduct in the interview. He also suggests some indications for occasional therapist self-disclosure. These include enhancing the patient's reality testing, the provision of interpersonal feedback, increasing the patient's self-esteem, promoting identification with the therapist, and resolving certain transference resistances.

GUIDELINES FOR STUDENTS

With this brief review of some of the issues involved in self-disclosure, I propose a few very general guidelines for making a decision to disclose personal material:

1) The therapist can be genuine and be himself or herself in the course of psychotherapy without disclosing highly personal material.

2) The more personal the material the therapist considers disclosing, the greater the need to consider carefully the reasons for the proposed disclosure.

3) The more urgently the therapist feels a need to disclose, the greater the need to consider carefully the reasons for the proposed disclosure.

4) The most common therapist's disclosure is sharing feelings with a patient about the patient's communications in order to provide interpersonal feedback regarding the pa-

tient's impact on others. This may be a particularly useful form of intervention with patients whose projections to others play a prominent role in their difficulty.

5) Certain patients with severe and chronic psychopathology and for whom treatment goals are limited may be helped by considerable therapist's disclosure, if it is not highly personal. For some of these patients, the once or twice monthly therapy sessions may represent rare moments of relief from alienation and loneliness.

6) When the therapist experiences intense feelings in the psychotherapy sessions that cannot be hidden and the patient notes them, they should not be denied.

7) On some occasions, major outside events will influence the therapist's feelings and may be disclosed under these circumstances.

8) Errors on the part of the therapist should be acknowledged.

9) No disclosure should be made without giving consideration to the most probable impact on the patient.

These directions reflect very general guidelines to the beginner who, at early stages of training, has not had the time to master the complex observational skills and theoretical framework necessary to consider quickly the interplay of variables involved in making a decision about self-disclosure. As psychotherapists gain experience, their clinical judgment increases and the need for general guidelines lessens. Some of the trainees move toward a classical psychoanalytic neutrality with its clear and generally negative stance on self-disclosure. Others move toward the existentialist position with its greater opportunity for self-disclosure. As teachers, our concern is to provide a better start for young therapists.

TRAINING EXPERIENCES

The seminar has no specific exercises for learning self-disclosure as an intervention technique. Throughout the audiovisual exercises and the later interviews with hospitalized patients, however, the complex issue of self-disclosure is discussed repeatedly as it applies in different contexts. The initial emphasis is on the student's (understandable) tendency to remain hidden by adopting a distant and stereotyped professional role. This is discouraged, and the students are encouraged to allow themselves to be more genuinely themselves in the interviews. They are told that showing interest and concern is an appropriate stance for therapists. As they experiment with a more natural style in the exercises, it becomes important for them to learn how much they may disclose without any awareness of the disclosure. Becoming aware of indirect disclosure is frequently painful because it often reveals the student's underlying anxiety. Commonly, this discomfort is exposed by the therapist's sudden change of subject, interview form, or even posture during an interview. Such anxiety is clearly reflected in the following example from an interview with a "patient" (actress) who is behaving seductively with a male, first-year resident.

> *Therapist*: . . . and after your boyfriend broke up with you how did you feel?
> *Patient*: Lousy.
> *Therapist*: Tell me more about it.
> *Patient*: Well, at first hurt and sad—then pissed off. After a few weeks I got horny (she stretches her legs towards his chair and rubs her thigh).
> *Therapist*: . . . hurt . . . and sad and then angry . . .
> *Patient*: . . . and horny.
> *Therapist*: (Leans far back in his chair) . . . well . . . perhaps . . . I . . . let's move on to some questions about . . . your family. Where were you born?

This student experienced significant anxiety as the result of the "patient's" seductiveness. He was uncertain about what to do —and switched the subject to a more structured form of interviewing with which he felt safer. In doing so, he disclosed his underlying anxiety. In his discussion following the review of the videotaped interview, he shared openly with the group his fear of the woman's seductiveness and his own sexual arousal during this stage of the interview.

Several of the initial audiotaped stimuli involve patients con-

fronting or questioning the therapist directly. In some, the focus
of the confrontation is the patient's perception of the here-and-
now of the therapeutic relationship. Others, however, deal with
an aspect of the therapist's private life. Beginning therapists
often find these to be very difficult exercises. They are introduced
to the concept that questions from patients may not be requests
for information, but are really vehicles for expressing other concerns. Many of the confrontations sound hostile and attacking—
"What about you? I hear you're getting a divorce . . .?" The students are encouraged to consider the possibility that it may be
more helpful to attempt to deal with the underlying concern than
it is to answer the question. The issue, however, can be more painful when the patient's confrontation involves the here-and-now
of the therapeutic relationship. This, too, may represent a host
of other concerns, but usually requires that the therapist not evade
the apparent substantive issue. This is necessary, both because the
relationship itself is central to the work of therapy and also because the therapist must discriminate between transference issues
and astute observations on the part of the patient. In this exploration, there may be a need for the therapist to disclose his or her
feelings about the state of the relationship clearly. It is important
for all patients to have their perceptions of interpersonal reality
validated or refuted, but it is of particular importance for severely
disturbed patients who commonly distort, misperceive, and project. Responding directly to the patient's observations may
occasion self-disclosure on the part of the therapist. This rarely
involves intimate material, and usually it can be handled by acknowledging the patient's perceptiveness or misperception. Such
a level of self-disclosure may facilitate rather than interfere with
the patient's exploration.

Carkhuff's (12) scale for the measurement of self-disclosure is
studied by the students. In this scale, we find an attempt to
operationalize the range or levels of therapist self-disclosure that
most often are associated with existential psychiatry. At low
levels, the therapist is presented as detached, disinterested, and
ambiguous. This reflects, I believe, confusion about the issue of
self-disclosure. A therapist may, and should, communicate in-

volvement, interest, and clarity without raising the question of self-disclosure. At somewhat higher, but still non-facilitative, levels of self-disclosure, the therapist answers questions, but does not volunteer personal information. I have referred earlier to the fact that questions from patients often are not simple requests for information, and to handle them as if they were may reflect a naive perception. At the level of minimum facilitation, the therapist is described as disclosing his or her reactions to the patient. At high levels, however, the scale suggests that the therapist is involved in volunteering intimate and detailed material "in keeping with the helpee's needs." There are no guidelines with which to measure or evaluate how the disclosure meets the patient's needs or which needs are met. The seminar does not propose this position for beginning therapists because it represents a polar position unsupported by either clinical experience or adequate research documentation. I make this point with some emphasis because I feel that in regard to some other variables involved in the psychotherapeutic transactions, Carkhuff presents useful training exercises for beginning therapists.

As the seminar moves into the stage where the students interview patients behind a one-way screen, attention turns to the therapist's impact upon the interview process. Although this issue is discussed in some detail in Chapter 6, which focuses on the therapist's need to develop an awareness of the interaction in which he or she is participating, a few comments appear appropriate at this time. It is obvious that a therapist discloses a great deal about himself or herself in many ways. He does so even when he does not consciously intend to. His appearance, mannerisms, style of speech, and posture, along with other individual characteristics, provide the patient with many clues about the therapist. Often, patients scan intensely for such clues because they need to feel accepted, safe, and certain. An initial goal of training beginning therapists is to help them develop an awareness of the ways in which their personal characteristics affect patients. Without this awareness, a therapist is unable to evaluate responses to his person that may reflect important aspects of the patient's dilemma. Often, it is considered that this type of awareness can come about only through personal therapy or psychoanalysis. The seminar provides a complementary source of learning for the beginning students. It has a particular power because much of the feedback to the individual student comes from peers in the seminar.

The second basic task involves the students in becoming more sensitive to the multiple ways they each communicate anxiety within the interview. This type of disclosure is very real, readily identified by the student's peers, probably noted and responded to by some patients, and frequently comes with some degree of surprise to the individual student.

The third objective of the seminar is to provide the students with information about the widely different positions of the various schools regarding self-disclosure and to encourage them not to adopt an extreme position at an early stage of their training. Rather, they are presented with the very general guidelines introduced in this chapter and encouraged to take a conservative position as regards disclosing highly personal material. The essence of this approach is that the introduction of these crucial issues early in the career of psychotherapists provides them an opportunity to experience their complexities. Gradually, as psychotherapists mature and develop increasing clinical judgment, there is perhaps less need for this type of structure. Although learning to reveal themselves comfortably and helpfully inevitably involves pain for beginners, the structure—both theoretical and experiential—provides support and is seen as superior to dropping the novices into the deep end of the pool and watching their frantic, "stay-alive" maneuvers. Self-disclosure is one of the more anxiety-filled aspects of psychotherapy for students, and the absence of clear guidelines makes learning a difficult experience. When students discuss this difficulty in the seminar, I must respond that we don't know with certainty; that process research is inconclusive; and that it is to be hoped that their generation of therapists will improve our understanding of complicated issues like the role of therapist's self-disclosure in effective psychotherapy.

REFERENCES

1. WEINER, M., *Therapist Disclosure: The Use of Self in Psychotherapy.* Boston: Butterworth Publisher, to be published, 1978.
2. NAMNUM, A., "Activity and Personal Involvement in Psychoanalytic Technique." *Bulletin of the Menninger Clinic,* Vol. 40:2, March, 1976, pp. 111-112.
3. GREENSON, R. R., "Beyond Transference and Interpretation." *International Journal of Psychoanalysis,* 53:213-217, 1972.
4. HAVENS, L. L., "The Existential Use of the Self." *American Journal of Psychiatry,* 131:1, 1-10, January, 1974.
5. JOURARD, S. M., and RESNICK, J. L., "Some Effects of Self-Disclosure Among College Women." *Journal Humanistic Psychology,* 10:84-93, 1970.
6. LIEBERMAN, M. A., YALOM, I. D., and MILES, M. D., *Encounter Groups: First Facts.* New York: Basic Books, 1973.
7. WEINER, M. F., CODY, V. D., and ROSSON, B., "Studies of Therapist and Patient Affective Self-Disclosure." *Group Process,* 6:27-42, 1974.
8. KANGAS, J. A., "Group Members' Self-Disclosure: A Function of Preceding Self-Disclosure by Leader or Other Group Member." *Comp. Group Studies,* Feb., 1971.
9. TRUAX, C. B., and CARKHUFF, R. R., *Toward Effective Counseling and Psychotherapy: Training and Practice.* New York: Aldine, 1967.
10. WEINER, M. F., Timberlawn Foundation Guest Lectureship, April, 1977.
11. SEARLES, H. F., *Collected Papers on Schizophrenia and Related Subjects.* New York: International Universities Press, 1965.
12. CARKHUFF, R. R., *Helping and Human Relations,* Vol. I, 208-209. New York: Holt, Rinehart & Winston, Inc., 1969.

CHAPTER 5

+++

Skills of Detachment

+++

++

The balance of intimacy and detachment has been considered
thus far primarily on the side of increasing students' capacities
for intimacy. The role of the therapist's detachment, the other
half of the balance, is also seen differently by the major schools
of psychotherapy. The objective-descriptive, psychoanalytic, and
interpersonal schools emphasize the therapist's capacity for detachment in order to observe, correlate, synthesize, and construct
hypotheses that are involved in the formulation of the patient's
dilemma and whatever treatment strategies the therapist enter-
tains. As Havens (1) has pointed out, the objective-descriptive
school is concerned centrally with the patient's signs and symptoms; the psychoanalytic school with the content of the patient's
mental life, resistance, and transference; and the interpersonal
school with the patient's projections to the therapist and the
maneuvers of the therapist to counter or prevent such projections.

These differences in the three schools regarding the nature of the data collected do not negate the fact that each school emphasizes that one role of the therapist is to be a more-or-less detached expert.

The existential school, however, in its central emphasis on being and staying, eschews any attempt at detached objectivity. "In the effort to project one's self into the other, every preconception that the patient might match is excluded. If we 'recognize' the patient, we have lost him. We are to keep looking for the person, not for something that relates to our own ideas"(2). Forming a judgment or reaching a conclusion is a temptation the existential therapist must avoid, for to succumb takes away the patient's uniqueness. In this way, the existential school is not only radical, but differs sharply from the other three schools.

As noted earlier, the seminar proposes a balance of intimacy and detachment, and it is the intent of this chapter to describe those exercises designed to increase the students' skills in the techniques that are more detached. Beginning therapists must learn six basic skills that come to form the foundation of this part of their expertise. These are the ability: 1) to listen for associations; 2) to identify major themes and affects; 3) to recognize signs of conflict or increased arousal; 4) to identify mechanisms of defense; 5) to observe nonverbal behavior; and 6) to construct a clinical formulation.

ASSOCIATIONS

A psychotherapist follows the train of the patient's associaitons and, in the process, notes linkages between various areas of mental content. This type of listening, derived from psychoanalysis, has become a central part of most psychotherapies. It is through recognizing associative links that the therapist constructs hypotheses about the patient's unconscious needs and conflicts. It is a type of psychotherapeutic activity that is cognitive and requires the therapist to observe the patient objectively at some interpersonal distance. The therapist may use a variety of techniques to facilitate the patient's flow of associations.

This type of verbal activity by the patient also brings repressed affects and early memories to the surface and provides the therapist a more-or-less spontaneous piece of patient verbal behavior. Recognition of the formal characteristics of that verbal behavior may provide valuable insight into certain patient characteristics. Weintraub and Aronson (3, 4, 5, 6, 7, 8, 9) have called attention to patterns of responses and characterized a variety of psychopathological conditions by their use of negators, qualifiers, retractors, and evaluators. Compulsive, neurotic patients (3), for example, reveal increased use of negators, retractors, evaluators, and explainers. These researchers then relate these formal verbal characteristics to the processes of denial (negators), undoing (retractors), heightened superego functions (evaluators), and rationalization (explainers). Gottschalk and his coworkers (10) have studied also the patterns of speech of psychiatric patients, and their findings provide the therapist with data useful in understanding the patient.

The ability to encourage a patient's spontaneous verbalization and to follow the trains of associations produced is an important psychotherapeutic skill. Students are encouraged to note the links in associations, the emergence of previously repressed affects and memories, and the formal mechanisms in the speech of their patients. The early structured exercises in the seminar, for the most part, do not provide the students with adequate material for this type of learning because they are limited, two-part interchanges (patient statement-student response). This psychotherapeutic skill is introduced at the point in the seminar when actual patients are interviewed behind a one-way screen. The skill is discussed, and subsequently one of the students is assigned to observe the interview and to monitor and record the patient's associations in writing. During the discussion period following the interview, he reports his observations to the group. The group quickly becomes intrigued by linkages and jumps in the patient's verbalizations which seem to be relatively independent of the interviewer and context and, as such, may reflect unconscious associations.

More often than not, the students are fascinated by this aspect of learning. In addition to the intrinsic fascination that unconscious processes hold for all of us, I believe there are other factors that go into the students' enthusiasm. So much of the seminar up to this point in time has focused on the therapist—his or her responses, anxieties, and empathic capacities—that they are relieved to shift the focus of their observation to the patient. This is familiar terrain, and during such activity they can be detached and expert detectives.

It is at this point that the instructor must deal with the students' tendency to close prematurely. Many students rush to some type of diagnostic conclusion on the basis of very little data. It is important to present a model of tentativeness and to discuss openly how often each of us moves to premature closure about a patient, and then attends only data consistent with that initial impression.

RECOGNIZING MAJOR THEMES AND AFFECTS

Listening for associations has, as one of its primary functions, the study of the linkages between themes in the patient's productions. There is often, however, a major theme, or perhaps several major themes, in most interviews. Examples of a major theme might be a particular need of the patient's, a certain relationship pattern, or a particular period of the patient's life. "More than anything else, what is the patient trying to examine or discuss with the interviewer?" is the question posed by the instructor. Even after a group discussion of the associative material, it is surprising how many differences of opinion the group members may have about the major theme or themes. It is as if the inference necessary to come to a decision about the major theme allows each student to process the associative material idiosyncratically. It is helpful to have each group member write what he sees as the major theme. There is usually some agreement, but several of the group may report a different theme as central to the interview. Most often, this appears to represent a failure to include in the synthesis one area of the interview that arouses fears in the therapist, who then focuses on aspects of the interview that are tangential to what most members of the group perceive as the major theme.

The students are asked also to consider what they have observed to be the major affective state of the patient. There is generally more agreement about the major affect, and the group moves quickly to identifying different levels or intensities of the emotions. For example, "Although the patient's anger is the predominant affect, there is an underlying sadness apparent." It is helpful to request the student to present the observations leading to these judgments. This is particularly necessary when the student suggests an "underlying" affect because of the tendency to perceive as subtle affects those states suggested by psychodynamic theory. The students learn to note facial expressions, changes in vocal characteristics, and other signs that are presumptive evidence of less intense, masked, or underlying affective states.

RECOGNIZING CONFLICT OR INCREASED AROUSAL

There are moments in most interviews when the patient manifests evidence of conflict or increased affective arousal. Often this is so marked as to be obvious to all, but, on other occasions, the evidence is subtle and fleeting. The evidence itself can take many forms—a sudden change in the tempo or intensity of the patient's speech, an unusual body movement or postural change, signs of sudden autonomic nervous system activity, such as blanching, blushing, or perspiration, or unusual word usage or metaphoric communication (11). The seminar attempts to increase the beginning therapist's sensitivity to these messages. This type of observational skill is introduced when the participants begin to interview patients behind the one-way screen. One observer is assigned the task of monitoring the interview for clues to deeper, hidden emotions (what have come to be called "tips of the iceberg"). Following the interview, the student reports these observations to the group, and they discuss both the meaning of the signs and whether or not the interviewer noted them and chose to invite the patient to explore. Occasionally, there is disagreement within the group about whether or not a particular patient's behavior reflects a patient's feelings or an understandable, interactional response to something the interviewer is communicating.

MECHANISMS OF DEFENSE

The students' increasing sensitivity to the patient's associations, major themes and affects, and clues to hidden affects leads the

seminar to a focus on psychological mechanisms of defense. To
develop awareness about the defense mechanisms of another person with whom one is interacting is both complex and difficult.
The observational skills discussed up to this point—following
associations, recognizing major themes and affects, and identifying clues to hidden affect—involves a lesser degree of inference.
For the most part, they reflect a type of perceptual awareness;
they stick close to the sensory data. Although one must be alert
to the multiple ways in which the interviewer may influence what
the patient says, such observations are based upon the facilitation
of as free and spontaneous speech as possible. However, identifying another's psychological defenses requires a much greater level
of inference, and there is greater opportunity for error. In particular, it is easy to note only that which fulfills one's early presumptions about the patient.

A more active error occurs when the interviewer establishes a
certain type of interaction with the patient (for example, cognitive) and then labels the patient's responses to the interviewer's
cues as "the patient's pathological defenses." Because the seminar
focuses early on affect, the student might identify a patient's
responses to a cognitive interview as "avoidance of affect," "denial
of affect," or "intellectualization." For example, a first-year resident interviewing a young woman reintegrating from a psychotic
episode was involved in the following interchange:

> *Patient*: . . . and then my mother died.
> *Interviewer*: What happened?
> *Patient*: She was killed in an accident.
> *Interviewer*: Tell me about it.
> *Patient*: She lost control of her car and skidded into a ravine.
> *Interviewer*: You were how old at that time?
> *Patient*: Nine.
> *Interviewer*: What else do you remember about it?
> *Patient*: . . . oh . . . just . . . it was very bad.
> *Interviewer*: Who took care of you?
> *Patient*: My grandparents.
> *Interviewer*: Anything else that comes to mind about it?
> *Patient*: No.

The interviewer, in his summary to the group, described the patient as using denial of affect and intellectualization. He appeared unaware of the way his questions and responses invited the patient to avoid exploring her feelings about the loss of her mother. The group pointed out his part in the exchange, and the group member recording the patient's associations read the student the segment reproduced above. The student quickly acknowledged how effectively he had prevented the patient from exploring her feelings about the loss and how unaware of it he had been at the time. He related that his own father had died several years earlier, and he wondered if his own feelings about that loss had prevented his encouraging the patient to explore his feelings.

It might be useful to illustrate the way the interchange could have evolved that might have led to the recognition of a patient's denial of affect and intellectualization.

> *Patient*: . . . and then my mother died.
> *Interviewer*: That must have been tough.
> *Patient*: She was killed in an accident.
> *Interviewer*: It was a difficult time for you . . .
> *Patient*: She lost control of her car and skidded into a ravine.
> *Interviewer*: How did you feel?
> *Patient*: I was nine at the time.
> *Interviewer*: Can you get at what you felt at the time?
> *Patient*: My grandparents took care of me.

In this illustration, the interviewer repeatedly invites the patient to explore and share the feelings involved in the loss of his mother. The patient's apparent inability to do so raises for the interviewer the question of the patient's denial of affect and use of intellectualization. The issue of the patient's use of these defenses can be considered legitimately in this interchange because the interviewer invited affect and did not avoid it as occurred in the first interchange.

Although the participants learn rapidly about the pitfalls of the "invite-then-label" process, they continue to struggle with the complex task of identifying defense mechanisms during the interview. Vaillant (12) states that we observe behavior and infer defenses, that defenses are easier to talk about than to validate consensually, are recognizable only in the extent to which they distort events we can see, are essentially processes rather than events and, as such, are intrinsically difficult to define. Although these observations do not help in the task of identifying discrete mechanisms of defense, they are most useful as an orienting structure for the beginning therapist. Vaillant presents clinical data that support the concept of a hierarchy of ego mechanisms of defense. At the most primitive level are the narcissistic defenses which include delusional projection, psychotic denial, and distortion. These defenses are common before age five and in adult dreams and fantasies. They alter reality, and appear "crazy" to the observer.

Immature defenses—projection, schizoid fantasy, hypochondriasis, passive-aggressive behavior, and acting out—are common in "healthy" individuals* ages 3 to 16, and in character and affective disorders. Vaillant suggests that they are used to alter distress engendered either by the threat of interpersonal intimacy or the threat of experiencing its loss. (They might occur, therefore, in the process of intensive psychotherapy, with its particular kind of intimacy.) To an observer, the immature defenses most often appear as socially undesirable behavior.

Neurotic defenses (at a healthier level of behavior) include intellectualization, repression, displacement, reaction formation, and dissociation. They are seen in neurotic disorders, and to some degree in "healthy" individuals age 3 to 90, and in mastering acute stress. Their primary use is in altering private feelings or instinctual expression; to an observer, they appear to be only individual quirks.

In Vaillant's framework, mature defenses include altruism, humor, suppression, anticipation, and sublimation. They are common in "healthy" individuals aged 12 to 90. Vaillant likens them to well-orchestrated composites of simpler mechanisms considered by some to be so "nearly conscious" as not to be defenses, but coping mechanisms. They integrate conscience, reality, interper-

---

* There are contrary data (13, 14) which suggest that these mechanisms are not seen in normal adolescents.

sonal relationships, and private feelings and, to the observer, they appear as convenient virtues.

Vaillant's hierarchy helps the beginning therapist to deal with clusters of mechanisms and to think in terms of levels of adaptive competence. It does not purport to provide clues to the identification of defense mechanisms from interview material. The students are encouraged to provide a situation that is optimal for the patient's exploration and to monitor their own impact constantly. It is in the patient's failure to explore under highly facilitative conditions that defenses (resistances to exploration) can best be noted. The resistances, if repeated and enduring, may then be dealt with directly by confrontation and clarification.

Another valuable source of learning is in the work of MacKinnon and Michels (15). These writers have presented a format for the interview which emphasizes the influence of the patient's psychopathology on the interview process. They describe the common psychodynamics of most clinical entities (that is, the hysteric, depressive, phobic, etc.) and the ways in which patients with such disturbances defend against exploration. Students are usually enthusiastic about the material presented by these authors. At the same time, its attractiveness and cohesiveness raise the question of how much information is sufficient. The data are frequently elusive in nature, and there is danger of premature closure. It is in the tremendous pull to see patients simplistically —only as the bearers of certain psychodynamic constellations— that the beginner can most often miss both the patient's uniqueness and the therapist's impact on the patient's behavior. For those reasons, the introduction of psychodynamic material into the seminar must be done in a way that emphasizes the complexity of the basic observational data upon which the psychodynamic inferences rest.

NONVERBAL BEHAVIOR

Attention to the patient's nonverbal behavior begins early in the seminar, during the use of videotaped patient stimuli statements. The initial emphasis is on facial expressions, but quickly includes postural messages and body movements. A helpful exercise is for the group to watch videotaped or filmed interviews without the sound and to make observations about affective messages.

As the participants begin to interview patients, one observer is assigned the task of monitoring the nonverbal behavior of both the patient and the interviewer. In reporting to the group, he or she distinguishes between those nonverbal behaviors of the patient that appear directly responsive to messages from the interviewer and those that seem unrelated to the behavior of the interviewer. Although there is ample evidence of both, the interviewer is surprisd how often nonverbal behavior of the patient appears to the group to be responsive to the interviewer's messages and cues—"the nonverbal ballet." The emphasis is placed on the awareness of behavior that the therapist encourages, and the tendency to (mis)interpret it as coming entirely from the patient.

The students find the work of Scheflen (16, 17) to be helpful as an orienting structure. His emphasis on the contextual correlates of postural changes has been particularly exciting to them, and they incorporate this knowledge into their observations of each other. Scheflen's intriguing work on quasi-courtship behavior has provided the students with an additional conceptual tool. "Did you notice the patient's smoothing her dress? Did you think she was quasi-courting, searching for contact with you?" is the type of use made of this concept. The members of the group are also sensitive to their own comparable behavior and attempt to relate it to some momentary sense of having lost contact with the other.

The students provide each other with considerable feedback about each individual's characteristic, nonverbal language. One male student consistently moved his head closer to individuals he talked to than the others preferred. This tendency to intrude into the space around others was something of which this student was unaware until his colleagues pointed it out to him. Another student rubbed his thigh as he listened intently to the patients he interviewed. The group was able to help him see that such behavior gave the patient an ambiguous and often threatening erotic message. A young woman student was not aware of her unusually rigid posture, and the group helped her to see its impact as a message that the interaction was formal and distant.

Teaching the beginning therapists to listen for associations, to identify major themes and affects, to recognize clues to deep affect, to identify mechanisms of defense, and to recognize non-verbal messages has several purposes. First, it is a structured and, in part, experiential type of learning that will continue throughout the students' training period and, hopefully, throughout their entire psychotherapeutic careers. A major source of continued learning in these areas is individual supervision.

A second purpose of this aspect of the seminar is to teach the students a systematic approach to collecting data to be used in constructing hypotheses about the patient. The students are encouraged to construct a hypothesis after each exploratory interview behind the one-way screen, and one participant is given this responsibility. Although the tentativeness of the hypothesis is emphasized, the instructions are to pull together and synthesize the observations into a clinical formulation.

CONSTRUCTION OF A CLINICAL FORMULATION

After the completion of the interview and discussion of the interviewer's conduct of the interview based upon the interview variables each observer has been monitoring, the group considers the question, "What did we learn about the patient?" It is convenient to have a blackboard available and for the instructor to lead the students' initial efforts to synthesize their observations. The instructor poses a series of questions starting with the patient's mental content as reflected in the associations and the major themes. There is often evidence that suggests the presence of a central conflict, but, whether the major mental content is seen as theme or conflict, it is the starting point for the clinical formulation.

Next to be considered and noted briefly on the blackboard is the major affect. An example is, "A young man who is intensely conflicted about closeness and appears to be very sad."

Then the patient's use of certain defenses is summarized. In this instance, they might include schizoid fantasy, projection, displacement, repression, and intellectualization. The group would note if there were immature defenses in addition to the more common and less discriminating neurotic level defenses.

Next in the order of consideration are whatever historical and symptom-oriented data were obtained in the exploratory interview. The young man in this example had discussed using speed intravenously for several years. He had talked about his mother's death after a long illness when he was nine and his father's alcoholism during the same period of his life.

At this point, the members of the group shared their diagnostic considerations, agreeing that the young man was neither psychotic nor classically neurotic, but that he did have a serious personality disturbance with an associated addiction to amphetamines. The tentativeness of the diagnostic consideration was emphasized, and the discussion turned to treatment. The students were asked to describe the patient's ego strengths, and they noted his apparent intelligence and the suggestion in the exploratory interview that he had some capacity for self-exploration, evidence of ability to observe himself (observing ego functions), and some conscious motivation to change. The students felt that the patient was likeable; most of their fantasies about him involved the notion of a sad and lonely little boy who both desperately desired, and was fearful of, closeness.

Pulling the group's observations together in this way results in a beginning hypothesis about the patient's dilemma. Although the instructor emphasizes that subsequent interviews almost always yield data that modify the early hypothesis, he or she stresses that the professional therapist does have the responsibility to bring the observations together and construct a tentative hypothesis.

At this point, the resident involved in the patient's care in the hospital shares with the group the clinical data accumulated during inpatient care. This includes the results of a lengthy social history, ward observations, psychological testing, and other traditional data sources. Most often, the observations growing out of the 25-minute exploratory interview are congruent with the results of the more detailed and intensive clinical workup, but frequently there are aspects of the patient's difficulty that were not apparent in the exploratory interview (for example, several brief, psychotic episodes during the past year).

The students' early experiences in the seminar with this type of clinical formulation bring into focus two problems that, to some degree, will occupy them throughout their careers. The first, of course, is the balance of intimacy and detachment required of the therapist. The act of formulating the patient's dilemma highlights for the beginner that behavior is understandable, and there is excitement and, perhaps, a sense of newfound power in the ability to recognize underlying themes, defenses, and syndromes. The student often experiences a potent pull to a role model characterized by detachment. This underscores the existentialists' position that once a therapist begins to compare, contrast, and conclude about a patient, the capacity for being with him or her deeply is diminished. This pull is augmented by the therapist's feeling of security in the detached position: He or she is the expert at some distance from the patient who, more often than not, is seen as very different.

The instructor's belief that at different moments during the interview a therapist is either deeply with the patient at a feeling level or is in a more detached and cognitive position needs repeated emphasis at this point. Greenson's (18) psychoanalytic perspective is helpful in the reiteration of this crucial issue. Rangell (19) states that objective listening is the imperishable core of the psychoanalytic method and adds, "The maintenance of a proper blend, of the indispensable analytic position fused with the necessary clinical, empathic, and intuitive skills for an optimum conduct of the therapeutic process, remains the most subtle task to achieve and develop . . ." (p. 93).

Strupp (20) underscores not only the need for both the detached, technical skills and the subjective use of self, but also the need to keep them separate in one's mind. He states, "As long as the clinician can separate and clearly keep apart the subjective and objective elements in his operations, he is able to function appropriately and (assuming he has the necessary training and experience) adequately in the clinical role. It is when the two segments interact in unknown and unconscious ways that the interest of the patient may be served less well. The perpetual problem with which the clinician is faced at every juncture in his work is . . . to be able to distinguish what is within himself and what is within the patient, and to know the difference."

A second problem associated with the therapist's skills that require more detachment—data collection and clinician formulation—concerns the therapist's tendency to close his or her collection of data prematurely. Elstein and co-workers (21) have presented a preliminary theory of the medical inquiry that is the basis for their studies of the reasoning process of expert physicians. I feel that their work is a particularly significant commentary on the reasoning processes of the psychotherapist in the attempt to formulate impressions of the patient's situation. Their theory asserts that physicians generate specific diagnostic hypotheses well before they have gathered sufficient data. They state (p. 89), ". . . the experienced physician appears to leap directly to a small array of provisional hypotheses very early in his encounter with the patient." The hypotheses come out of the physician's background knowledge precipitated by early observations of the patient. Four components of generating hypotheses are described: 1) attending to initially available clues; 2) identifying problematic elements from among the clues; 3) associating from the problematic elements to long-term memory and back, generating hypotheses and suggestions for further inquiry; and 4) informally ranking the hypotheses. Factors that influence the ranking of hypotheses include their statistical likelihood, seriousness, treatability, and novelty. The authors state that following the generation and rough rank-ordering of the hypotheses, they are systematically tested in the "familiar medical workup." They suggest that the limits of human short-term memory could lead to rapid information overload if the hypotheses did not serve as data organizers.

I have experienced this process as they described it during those periods when I am thinking in a detached and objective way about my psychotherapy patients. It is also what occurs in case conferences when a consultant "thinks out loud" as the clinical data are presented. Elstein and his colleagues seem to have described with accuracy the basic format involved in clinical reasoning, and I think that it is applicable to the process of a psychiatric clinical formulation.

If there is validity in my impression, their description of the process emphasizes the dangers of the psychotherapist's premature closure. Elstein and his colleagues suggest that the systematic medical workup or search protects the clinician from the dangers inherent in generating hypotheses early. They note the difficulty most clinicians have in giving up an initial hypothesis if there is any confirmatory evidence for it. Hypotheses are necessary as an aid to search and memory, but one can make a strong commitment to an incorrect hypothesis unless one follows a systematic procedure that insures that one does not ask only those questions which tend to confirm an early hypothesis, and that one's inquiry provides an opportunity for data to emerge that could lead to alternate hypotheses. In my opinion, this reliance upon a more-or-less fixed system of inquiry is not characteristic of many skilled psychotherapists. There are, of course, some whose initial contacts with the patients are characterized by a meticulous history-taking, physical examination, and laboratory studies. Many, however, in the effort to meet the patient where he is, follow the leads the patient provides in a less directive and more collaborative manner. Some do both the less directive, collaborative interview and a detailed history in the same or several exploratory interviews. This is my suggestion to the residents in their initial contacts with patients with whom they may be involved in psychotherapy.

Nevertheless, to the extent to which we in psychiatry have no systematic approach to our investigation of the patient's situation, we are prone to premature closure and, on occasions, to serious defects in our understanding. This problem is introduced to the students and, although I have no completely satisfying solution, I am impressed with the need to have beginning therapists aware of the potential pitfalls involved in their more detached and objective thinking about their patients.

The skills and techniques which the therapist uses when he or she is "detached" are only introduced in this seminar. Much of the participants' subsequent training involves the acquisition and sharpening of these skills. In seminars, case conferences, the supervised care of patients and, in particular, individual psychotherapy supervision, the bulk of this learning occurs. These observational and synthesizing skills are introduced also by other faculty members in first-year courses focusing on the mental status examination, diagnostic systems, the psychiatric evaluation, and psychoanalytic theory. They have been added to this seminar after the early few years when the sole emphasis was on the importance of attending the patient's affect. I have come to appreciate more fully the importance of balancing those aspects of feelings (intimacy) with skills of detachment. Thus, the evolution of the seminar parallels some of my own changes. The seminar started with my personal dissatisfaction with therapy that appeared often to be too cognitive and detached. This led to the early focus on affective communication, empathy, and the therapist's use of his own feelings, memories, and fantasies in psychotherapy. After several years of an almost exclusive concern with the teaching and learning of the role of affect in psychotherapy, the seminar has moved to a central focus on the balance of intimacy and detachment.

There are others whose writings suggest concern with the training of therapists. I have been helped in particular by the reports of Muslin, Schlessinger, and Baittle (22, 23, 24) which have provided exciting ideas and innovative approaches to teaching.

Chessick's (25, 26) point that we know more than we teach applies equally to the affective and the cognitive aspects of psychotherapy. It is imperative that we translate that into teaching and exercises to provide students with a better base for beginning to be therapists than most of us experienced at early stages of our training.

REFERENCES

1. HAVENS, L. L., *Approaches to the Mind*. Boston: Little, Brown and Company, 1973.

2. HAVENS, L. L., "The Existential Use of the Self." *American Journal of Psychiatry*, 131:1, Jan. 1974, p. 2.

3. WEINTRAUB, W., and ARONSON, H., "The application of Verbal Behavior Analysis to the Study of Psychological Defense Mechanism: Methodology and Preliminary Report." *Journal of Nervous and Mental Disease*, Vol. 134, 169-181, 1962.

4. WEINTRAUB, W., and ARONSON, H., "The Application of Verbal Behavior Analysis to the Study of Psychological Defense Mechanisms, II: Speech Pattern Associated with Impulsive Behavior." *Journal of Nervous and Mental Disease*, Vol. 139, 75-82, 1964.

5. WEINTRAUB, W., and ARONSON, H., "The Application of Verbal Behavior Analysis to the Study of Psychological Defense Mechanisms, III: Speech Associated with Delusional Behavior." *Journal of Nervous and Mental Disease*, Vol. 141(2), 172-179, 1965.

6. WEINTRAUB, W., and ARONSON, H., "The Application of Verbal Behavior Analysis to the Study of Psychological Defense Mechanisms, IV: Speech Pattern Associated with Depressive Behavior." *Journal of Nervous and Mental Disease*, Vol. 141(1), 22-28, 1967.

7. WEINTRAUB, W., and ARONSON, H., "Application of Verbal Behavior Analysis to the Study of Psychological Defense Mechanisms, V: Speech Pattern Associated with Overeating." *Archives of General Psychiatry*, Vol. 21, 739-744, December, 1969.

8. ARONSON, H., and WEINTRAUB, W., "Sex Differences in the Verbal Behavior Related to Adjustive Mechanisms." *Psychological Rep.*, 21:965-971, 1967.

9. WEINTRAUB, W., and ARONSON, H., "Verbal Behavior Analysis and Psychological Defense Mechanisms, VI: Speech Pattern Associated with Compulsive Behavior." *Archives of General Psychiatry*, Vol. 30, 297-300, March, 1974.

10. GOTTSCHALK, L. A., and GLESSER, G. C., *Measurement of Psychological States.* University of California Press, 1969.

11. VOTH, H. M., "The Analysis of Metaphor." *Journal American Psychoanal. Association*, Vol. 18(3):599-621, July, 1970.

12. VAILLANT, G. E., "Theoretical Hierarchy of Adaptive Ego Mechanisms." *Archives of General Psychiatry*, Vol. 24, 107-118, February, 1971.

13. MASTERSON, J. F., *The Psychiatric Dilemma of Adolescence.* Boston: Little, Brown and Company, 1967.

14. OFFER, D., SABSHIN, M., and MARCUS, D., "Clinical Evaluation of Normal Adolescents." *American Journal of Psychiatry*, 121:864-872, 1965.

15. MACKINNON, R. A., and MICHELS, R., *The Psychiatric Interview in Clinical Practice.* Philadelphia: W. B. Saunders Company, 1971.

16. SCHEFLEN, A. E., "Quasi-Courtship Behavior in Psychotherapy." *Journal for the Study of Interpersonal Process*, 28:245-257, 1965.

17. SCHEFLEN, A. E., *A Psychotherapy of Schizophrenia: A Study of Direct Analyses.* Springfield, Illinois: Charles C Thomas, 1960.

18. GREENSON, R. R., "Empathy and Its Vicissitudes." *International Journal of Psychoanalysis*, 41:418-424, 1960.

19. RANGELL, L., "Psychoanalysis and the Process of Change." *International Journal of Psychoanalysis*, 87-98, 1975.

20. STRUPP, H. H., *Psychotherapy: Clinical, Research, and Theoretical Issues.* New York: Jason Aronson, Inc., 1973, p. 369.

21. ELSTEIN, A. A., KAGAN, N., SHULMAN, L. S., JASON, H., LOUPE, M. J., "Methods and Theory in the Study of Medical Inquiry." *Journal of Medical Education*, Vol. 47, February, 1972, pp. 85-92.
22. SCHLESSINGER, N., MUSLIN, H., and BAITTLE, M., "Teaching and Learning Psychiatric Observational Skills." *Archives of General Psychiatry*, Vol. 18, 549-552, May, 1968.
23. MUSLIN, H., and SCHLESSINGER, N., "Toward Teaching and Learning of Empathy." *Bulletin of the Menninger Clinic*, 35(4), pp. 262-271, July, 1971.
24. MUSLIN, H., "Clinical Exercises in Empathy." *Diseases of the Nervous System*, 35:8, 384-387, August, 1974.
25. CHESSICK, R. D., *How Psychotherapy Heals*. New York: Science House, 1969.
26. CHESSICK, R. D., *Why Psychotherapists Fail*. New York: Science House, 1971.

CHAPTER 6

++

Awareness of the Process

of the Interaction

++

In the effort to understand effective psychotherapy, research studies have focused on the patient, the therapist, and the treatment context. Using these variables, we continue to be unable to document the processes underlying successful psychotherapy. As a consequence, there is increasing interest in the process of the interaction between the therapist and patient.

Luborsky (1) has suggested the need to study the characteristics of the therapist-patient relationship, and has developed a rating procedure that permits the identification of two patterns of doctor-patient relationships—one that appears to be supportive and the other more collaborative. Strupp (2) discusses changing concepts in the therapist-patient relationship. He points out an increasing tendency to deal with the dynamics of the therapeutic situation in process terms with a greater emphasis on the here-and-now experience within the relationship. The traditional con-

117

cept of the therapist's objectivity has had to be reexamined because of increasing awareness that the information used in making objective judgments is filtered through and affected by the interaction between patient and therapist. Knight (3), in his paper on the therapeutic alliance, discusses a mutually observing relationship with a type of conjoint mental activity that can produce dyadic creativity. Although Knight's language is psychoanalytic, the constructs he refers to are clearly interactional rather than related to either therapist or patient individually.

Concurrently, with the increasing interest on the part of psychotherapy teachers and researchers in the interactional aspect of the psychotherapy (whether discussed as relationship or alliance), family systems researchers have identified interactional variables associated with different levels of family competence. Our own research group has reported findings from the study of healthy or competent families (4), and one of my colleagues, W. Robert Beavers (5), has spelled out that which such families may teach individual psychotherapists about promoting competence.

The suggestion that competent families have something to teach us about successful psychotherapy is based on the observation that both processes are involved centrally in nourishing individual competence. The competence of a family is judged, in part, by the degree to which it produces children who experience their own separateness and individuality and grow to personal autonomy. Although many patients enter psychotherapy for symptomatic relief, Beavers has articulated clearly that successful therapy involves personal growth with increased individuality and autonomy. These goals,* common to family and psychotherapy, led to the hypothesis that the interpersonal processes found to be essential to one may also characterize the other. Empirically, as well as theoretically, they provide us with a structure with which to assess the psychotherapeutic interaction.

---

* The other major goal or function of the family is the stabilization or maturation of the parental personalities. It is tempting, therefore, to wonder how much of psychotherapeutic process serves also this end for the therapist. This may suggest why many therapists, after moving on to other activities (for example, administration), continue to "see a few patients in therapy." At this stage of our knowledge, we should not minimize the personal benefits that may accrue to the helper.

First, however, let us review briefly the study of competent families. Families are studied in a variety of ways. The technique or approach that has the most intriguing implications for psychotherapy is best described as interactional. This approach studies the family as a system by providing the family with a problem to solve and examining the family's interactions (rather than the content of their exchanges) in solving problems. Rating scales are used to measure discrete variables involved in the relationship processes of the family as a whole.

In our study of families—both competent and dysfunctional—we have found that a group of specific, measurable variables correlate well with judgments regarding the overall level of competence of the family. One of the most significant variables is the distribution of overt power or interpersonal influence, which has predictable implications for the children. Healthy or competent families reveal clear patterns of shared parental power. Characteristically, the children in such families are not subjected to authoritarian use of parental power. We have described sharing of power in such families as demonstrating a pattern of leadership moving toward egalitarianism.

To pursue the analogy that psychotherapy is like a family, it is necessary to evaluate the therapist-patient interaction from the viewpoint of the way in which power is distributed between the two participants. Since patients come to a particular therapist because of the therapist's reputation and prestige, under most circumstances the relationship starts with the therapist having the bulk of the power. To share it with the patient, the therapist must insist that the relationship be a collaborative one in which what each thinks and feels is important. In this way, the responsibility for outcome is shared.

The model of shared and, if possible, equal power is one that may be misunderstood because of the differences in the roles of patient and therapist. The therapist has a knowledge of psychopathology, a theory of health and illness, an awareness of unconscious processes, and a variety of therapeutic skills. These determine his or her role as a professional, but do not mean that he or she is more powerful in the interaction, unless this knowledge and skill are utilized as controlling or indoctrinating forces.

A second variable from the study of competent families concerns both the efficiency of and the processes underlying their efforts to solve problems. Competent families are efficient problem-solvers; family members negotiate with each other to accomplish the task. It is this negotiation that has relevance for psychotherapeutic process. Competent families invite each member to participate, give careful consideration to the perceptions of each, and search for a consensus. Failing that, such families search for a compromise. It is in this reliance upon negotiation that competent families demonstrate clearly their commitment to shared power. Under ordinary circumstances, no single family member's view of reality dominates the group. We would study psychotherapeutic interactions, therefore, with an eye to how often the patient and therapist negotiate their different perceptions of a given event. It might be anticipated that therapist-patient relationships that are basically collaborative in nature would be characterized by high levels of negotiation.

A third and related variable concerns those processes noted in competent families that appear to encourage individual autonomy. This begins with a clear recognition of individual differences. This separateness is noted most in the degree to which individuals are asked to state openly their feelings and thoughts. At the same time, the competent family system has high levels of permeability. Members not only hear but they also acknowledge each other's feelings and thoughts. This clarity of expression and open acknowledgment without pressure for sameness or oneness is considered to be the basic interactional matrix in which individuality is nourished and autonomy may flourish.

In the psychotherapeutic interaction, we would look for comparable findings. How clear is each of the participants and, in particular, how much does the therapist invite open expression from the patient? How often is there clear acknowledgment of those findings and thoughts? Is the language of the therapist clear and specific or ambiguous and abstract?

A fourth group of variables concerns the competent family's

dealing with emotions. Such families are highly expressive of feelings—both positive and negative. There is a baseline mood of warmth and caring, liberally sprinkled with humor. Expressions of feelings (of any kind) usually evoke an empathic response. Conflict, when it evolves, is dealt with openly and immediately; there is nothing to suggest the long-smoldering, underlying conflicts found in dysfunctional families.

In the psychotherapeutic interaction, we would look for the way of encouraging expression of feelings and the level of empathic responsiveness of the therapist. We would anticipate that conflicts between the two participants would be dealt with early and with openness.

Beavers (5) has also discussed that which competent families can say to individual therapists about systems, contextual issues, and transcendent values. Although these issues are woven into the fabric of the seminar, the variables of power, task efficiency and negotiation, the encouragement of individual autonomy, and affect are more directly related to the study of psychotherapy as an interactional process.

THE THERAPIST'S IMPACT ON THE INTERACTION

There are two major tasks regarding the interaction that the seminar addresses. The first involves the efforts to increase the students' awareness of their impact upon the nature of the interaction. The second task involves the need for the therapist to monitor the interaction even though he or she is an active participant.

The therapist's ability to recognize his or her impact upon an interpersonal interaction in which he or she is participating is a continuous struggle throughout a lifetime of psychotherapeutic work. I believe that the difficulties this problem poses push some therapists to minimize the force of their own personalities and to develop a masked, underplayed therapeutic style. In doing so, they risk presenting a somewhat dehumanized model to the patient.

The most common pathway young therapists take to a clearer view of themselves is personal psychotherapy or psychoanalysis.

Chessick (6, 7) is among those who feel that all psychotherapists should involve themselves in either intensive psychotherapy or psychoanalysis. In our training program, most students enter personal therapy or psychoanalysis. A very few need to be told that they must do so in order to continue their development as therapists; most do so out of their own perceptions.

A psychotherapy training program has, I believe, the responsibility to encourage self-awareness in its students in as many ways as possible. In this seminar, a major focus is on the students' recognizing their own idiosyncratic perceptions and responses. By coming to understand the ways in which they perceive certain events idiosyncratically, the students begin to understand one aspect of their own impact on the interaction. This starts with the early exercises on cognitive empathy. Each student finds that a particular affect or area of content provokes some degree of perceptual difficulty. To recognize these highly individual difficulties is an early lesson for the beginning therapist.

The emphasis on warmth, respect, and genuineness early in training offers considerable opportunity for the beginner to learn about his or her impact on the interaction. In addition to the direct critique from the instructor and group regarding attitude, level of attentiveness, vocal characteristics, and nonverbal behavior, the student receives sensitive observations about any reduction in his or her usual levels of respect, warmth, and genuineness during certain interviews. The student learns that most frequently this means that something is bothering him or her about which he or she has been completely unaware—anxiety about the patient, a particular theme or affect within the interview, or perhaps even something in his or her personal life. Such knowledge of one's own impact is particularly valuable because, characteristically, it calls attention to aspects of one's person that have eluded awareness.

In a similar way, the focus on nonverbal behavior is instructive for the student. The observer monitoring this variable during interviews attends the nonverbal behavior of both the patient and therapist, and often describes the interactional aspects of the behavior. This nonverbal ballet occurs most often outside of the awareness of the interviewer and, although the interviewer may have noted the patient's nonverbal behavior, self-awareness is rare. Each student comes to an appreciation of the impact of his or her pattern of posture, movement, and facial expressiveness.

The Forced Fantasy Exercise is designed to promote increased awareness of each student's characteristic responses. In this experience, the group is shown a series of pictures depicting various affects, developmental stages, and human needs. There are ten pictures, including a nursing mother, children at play, a lonely, forlorn, neglected child, a nude woman, a nude man, an angry scene, and a person weeping at a graveside. Each student writes a fantasy incorporating the visual image. These are read aloud, and the group comments on each. Usually there is a common fantasy and several "deviant" fantasies. The students with deviant fantasies vary with each picture. The following are examples from a recent class of students:

One picture is of a young woman seated alone on a bench in a long, dark hall. Her head is forward and hangs down between her legs. The mood of the picture is almost always perceived as somber. The common fantasy contains the central theme of a woman alone and despondent—perhaps waiting in a courthouse hall. A first-year resident, a young, single woman, wrote a deviant fantasy seeing in the picture only a vase with a single rose in it. As she became aware of the extent of her deviance, she expressd shock and disbelief and asked to see the picture again. When it was projected, she went up to the screen and stared hard at the image. "I can see her now—but I would not have believed it." She went on to share with the group her own feelings of loneliness and the possible impact of those feelings on her perception and processing of the picture.

Another example from the same group of students involved a picture of children leaping from what appears to be a sand dune. They are perhaps nude—although that is difficult to determine because of shadows. The mood, however, is almost always seen as joyful and playful. This picture has a strong impact on fantasy formation, with most individuals responding with fantasies of being young, a child, and playing joyfully on the beach. Two first-year residents wrote deviant fantasies that were remarkably similar although the residents were seated apart. One, a young woman, wrote that these were children in another land—Africa, perhaps—who were running to escape a predator. The other resident wrote essentially the same fantasy, placing the fantasy in a different culture and without joy or play. In the discussion, both residents were amazed at their differences from the group. The young woman wondered if she had "seen" the picture differently because play had been absent from her childhood. She went on to describe growing up in a family where she was a "little adult" for as far back as she could recall. Her colleague, upon hearing this, indicated that he, too, had grown up with very little play. He was from a very religious family, and his childhood had been dominated by rules.

A major experience in learning about the therapist's impact on the therapeutic interaction occurs when each of the participants interviews the same actor "patient." These videotaped interviews are reviewed by the group, and the strikingly different interactions are noted. Some of the interviews go very well, and the actor may report having no sense of either acting or being on camera, but of having been caught up in an exploration of real, personal meaning. Other interviews go badly and result in the therapist's failure to establish contact, a resistant "patient," and an anxious, depressed interviewer. Although the pain is intense for students whose interviews have gone badly, the instructor and other participants offer both emotional support and specific criticism about the ways in which the interaction appeared to founder. Despite the risk to the students' self-esteem, this experience gives each student a rare opportunity to see himself or herself conduct an interview, brings the differences in therapist-"patient" interactions clearly into focus, and demonstrates the impact the interviewer can have upon the interaction.

As students are encouraged to learn about themselves and their impact on the therapist-patient interaction, they note an occasional tendency to label as pathology of the patient that which appears clearly evoked by the therapist. This is a theme running through the group's observations of each interview. For example, to encourage a patient to discuss an event in a cognitive way (what? how? when? why?), and then to see the patient as avoiding feelings by intellectualizing would prompt confrontation from the group.

In many ways, the students become sensitive to how a therapist may inadvertently influence the interaction. Learning about one's impact continues throughout training, and is a central function of individual supervision. The initial experiences in the seminar may have particular importance both because they occur early in training, and because they occur openly in front of the student's peers.

PROCESS OF THE INTERACTION

The skillful therapist has three constant sources of understanding which can be helpful to patients. He monitors the patients' associations, notes the resistances, observes nonverbal behavior, and perceives the patient in a variety of other sensory ways in the effort to be of maximum help. The therapist must also listen inwardly—to his or her own feelings, memories, and fantasies. A third source of understanding that is less readily appreciated is the process of the interaction itself. This type of meta-monitoring requires the therapist to observe an evolving process in which he or she is participating.

It is not possible to make the three observations at the same time. Beginning therapists in this seminar are encouraged to observe the process of the interaction from time to time during each interview. They are offered a format for making these observations which starts with the question, "What are the cadence, depth, and distance in this interaction?"

CADENCE

The cadence of the interaction is concerned both with who is doing the talking and the length of the speech sequences. A cadence in which the therapist makes brief statements that are followed by longer patient statements is called an exploratory cadence:

Therapist: . . . .
Patient: . . . .
Therapist: . . . .
Patient: . . . .
Therapist: . . . .
Patient: . . . .

Such a cadence suggests that exploration may be occurring although it does not guarantee it. It is considered a desirable cadence.

Two other types of cadence are noted. One involves the following pattern:

Therapist: . . . .
Patient: . . . . . .
Therapist: . . . .
Patient: . . . .
Therapist: . . . .
Patient: . . . . . .

This cadence suggests the presence of considerable resistance to exploration and, although there are times when it does not reflect resistance to exploration (periods of clarification, for example), its presence as the basic cadence of an interview is considered presumptive evidence of resistance to exploration.

Another type of cadence is the following:

Therapist: . . . .
Patient: . . . .
Therapist: . . . . . .
Patient: . . . .
Therapist: . . . .
Patient: . . . .

This pattern is the most difficult to evaluate because it may reflect resistance or quick but effective collaboration. Students become sensitive to the notion that if this pattern seems to dominate the interaction, they must be particularly attentive to the content in order to understand the implications of the cadence.

Cadence, then, is the first interactional process variable the students are asked to attend. It is an observational skill that generally gives the group little difficulty.

DEPTH OF EXPLORATION

An estimate of the depth of exploration occurring within the interaction is a more complex judgment. Essentially, the student is asked to consider whether therapist and patient maintain a focus and pursue its roots and ramifications, or rather tend to touch on a variety of areas superficially. Although interactions that fail to demonstrate exploration in depth have usually been considered as reflecting the patient's resistance, the students are taught to consider them as interactional phenomena until there is clear evidence that the therapist has made a maximum effort to facilitate deeper exploration. An interview lacking depth can be the result of the therapist's need to avoid a particular theme or affect.

INTERPERSONAL DISTANCE

The third aspect of the process of the interaction, the degree of interpersonal closeness or distance, concerns very inferential data. There is no reliable way to measure interpersonal distance, and we have only the impressions of the therapist and the group observing the interview. In practice, we consider that those interactions characterized by high levels of therapist's affective empathy demonstrate considerable closeness, and that those interactions characterized by the therapist's detached skills or interventions reveal greater interpersonal distance.

The students are instructed to listen to the language used by therapist and patient as a possible clue to interpersonal closeness and distance. If the language is abstract and formal, it is probable that interpersonal distance is greater than if the language is specific or concrete. Although Carkhuff (8) has suggested the importance of this variable as a therapist's characteristic, within the seminar it is used in regard to the language of both participants. Students are encouraged, of course, to use simple, specific, and concrete language and attempt in this way to encourage the patient to do likewise.

Kagan's (9) intriguing work with the Interpersonal Process Recall provides the group with a useful experience regarding interpersonal closeness and distance. In Kagan's technique, an interview is videotaped, following which one of the participants leaves the room and is replaced by a third person (the Inquirer). These two individuals review the videotape of the interview and their review is videotaped. The Inquirer stops the videotape of the initial interview whenever he or she sees something of interest (a sudden movement, change in voice characteristic, etc.) in either the interviewer or patient and attempts to explore with the participant what he or she was thinking or feeling at such moments. After 35-45 minutes of inquiry, the participant in the original interview leaves, and the inquiry is repeated with the other participant.

Kagan presents data to suggest that many clues in the interview (that were ignored) concern each participant's anxiety about how one is being perceived by the other. Apparently, both patient and therapist experience considerable concern about being accepted that is rarely talked about. The need for mutual acceptance seems to propel the participants closer together, and yet such closeness provokes anxiety in one or both of the participants. This can be reflected in fantasies of being devoured or losing one's individuality, and it leads to a rapid retreat in the form of increasing the interpersonal distance. Kagan suggests that throughout an interview, interpersonal closeness varies, propelled in one direction by the participants' need for acceptance, and in the other direction by the fear of closeness in one or both.

Kagan's provocative technique increases the students' appreciation of the importance of interpersonal closeness and distance as a characteristic of the interaction. It is time-consuming, but well worth the investment. Almost without exception, when the participants report what they were thinking but did not say during moments of unusual tension, their comments reflect the need for acceptance and fear of closeness. One example involved a student and his psychotherapy patient, both of whom volunteered for the Interpersonal Process Recall experiment. In the course of exploring with the patient (a young, attractive woman with a severe borderline syndrome) her feelings about the videotaping, she stated, "I'm not as comfortable as I am in your room." The resident quickly moved his hand to his mouth and reflected about the anxiety the videotape procedure provokes in everyone. In the subsequent Inquiry, the interview tape was stopped at this point and the patient discussed freely her spontaneous use of "room" rather than "office." Although she talked about sexual feelings, the major theme of her discussion was her strong desire for closeness. In the Inquiry with the therapist, he indicated that he heard her "slip" and felt it implied both a sexual and a more primitive type of closeness. His fantasy was of his getting up and leaving the recording studio. In this example, both the therapist and the patient were aware of, but ignored, the patient's slip of the tongue —and each had thoughts about its implications of sexuality and closeness—and talked of the more "comfortable" area, anxiety. Kagan's concept regarding the often unspoken theme of closeness was demonstrated strikingly.

The therapist's capacity to sense where the interaction is in terms of the level of interpersonal distance or closeness is a complex skill that involves not only knowing one's self in great depth, but also the ability to perceive subtle clues from the patient about the interactional process of moving toward or away from each other. Those interviews that are distinguished by a considerable sustained distance are easier for the therapist to recognize. As is true for other aspects of therapeutic skill, the concept of monitoring the interpersonal distance in the interaction can be introduced only; achieving a reasonable competence requires a much longer period of time. It is, perhaps, the task of a professional lifetime.

FOCUS

Another major area of learning about the process of the interaction involves the focus of the therapist-patient dialogue. The seminar teaches that the probability that effective work will be done in therapy is greatest when the focus is on the here-and-now of the ongoing relationship. Carkhuff (8) refers to this process as immediacy. Although he discusses it as something the therapist strives for or encourages, it can be considered an interactional focus that both participants share. It is the responsibility of the therapist, however, to encourage this focus when it seems appropriate.

This is a difficult area for beginning therapists because it is very different from interviewing with a focus on symptoms, the past, or another person. To explore with another what is happening "between us right now" seems like a perilous and anxiety-filled venture to most beginners. They are introduced to the concept early in the seminar when some of the stimuli in the exercises are directed at the here-and-now of the patient-therapist relationship. Later, as the students interview patients behind the one-way screen, there are multiple opportunities for the interviewer to encourage a focus on the here-and-now. Initially, these often concern their shared experience of being observed but, as the interview moves on, the students are encouraged to consider the possibility that *any* theme or affect of the patient may, in fact, reflect something of the here-and-now experience. ("As you describe how afraid of your father you've been, I find myself wondering if you're experiencing something like that here with me?") The students are encouraged also to move in the direction of a here-and-now focus any time the patient is discussing a person or situation of the same general order as the therapist or the interview. A patient's discussing doctors, a job interview, or an experience with a teacher should alert the therapist to the possibility that the patient may be communicating something about the here-and-now. An example from a student's interview follows. In this example, the student failed to encourage a needed focus on the here-and-now.

> *Therapist*: . . . and you felt afraid?
>
> *Patient*: Yes—I thought that I wouldn't get the job; it would be like all the other times.

Therapist: Another failure to feel accepted by someone important . . .

Patient: Exactly the same old story. I never seem to make it with people in authority.

Therapist: When did this all start?

In the discussion following this exchange, the student readily accepted the observation that he had repeatedly avoided a focus on the immediate. He wondered whether, in part, he was responding to the patient's physical unattractiveness and his own struggle to feel and be with someone who aroused his distaste.

The variables of cadence, depth, distance, and focus of the interaction can be thought of as orienting observations that tell one something of the basic process of the interaction. If we return to the family system variables mentioned earlier, it is possible to make observations that add substantially to our understanding of the interaction.

OVERT POWER

The degree to which a therapist shares the interpersonal influence and develops a collaborative relationship with the patient can be noted in a number of ways. First, how much does the therapist invite the patient's opinions about the meaning of a given event? Those therapists who make authoritarian interpretations are often operating out of a sense of great power. Those who are respectful of the patients' subjective perceptions of their own thoughts and ideas are often seen as sharing power. In a family, evidence of power is often reflected by an individual's asking repetitive, focused questions. In this way, he or she is able to constrict and mold the dialogue. In a similar manner, some therapeutic interactions are dominated by the therapist's relying on focused questions as the basic approach to dialogue. It is as if the therapist knows in advance where the interview should go. Focused questions have an appropriate function, but to rely on this form of dialogue in a major way raises serious questions about a therapist's ability to share power.

There are, of course, other ways in which one can sense the

distribution of power between patient and therapist, but these two—how often the patient's opinions are invited and how the therapist uses focused questioning—are easily available to the therapist in the attempt to monitor the process of the interaction.

NEGOTIATION AND TASK EFFICIENCY

Most inexperienced therapists have much to learn about the relevance of negotiation for the work of psychotherapy. In part, this may reflect their families of origin. Although there are no systematic data that speak directly to this issue, Henry et al. (10) suggest that many therapists come from dysfunctional families. If there is truth in that impression, many therapists did not learn negotiation as a primary approach to problem-solving as they grew up, and they may have carried a pattern of a dominant or powerful parent into their marriage. As the therapist grows and matures, he moves away from powerful "one-up" relationships toward relationships of more nearly equal power.

Negotiation and task efficiency are closely related to the way in which the therapist deals with his socially sanctioned power. The task of psychotherapy is to identify problems, explore them, and achieve solutions. Each therapist has occasional experiences in which psychotherapy wanders from its defined goal. When there is no continuity from session to session (although there may be a considerable sense of therapeutic encounter), there is little to suggest a joint commitment to the purpose of the process. Such observations about the therapist's interactions with patients are indicated when there is a sense of disquiet about where the therapy "is" and where it is "going." Too often, however, this phenomenon is considered only as evidence of the patient's resistance, without adequate consideration of its truly interactional nature.

ENCOURAGING AUTONOMY

The therapist who encourages his or her patient to become autonomous facilitates, first of all, the patient's sense of separateness and individuality. This is done by encouraging the patient to express feelings, thoughts, and ideas clearly. The therapist acknowledges and respects what the patient feels and thinks. In a comparable way, the therapist is clear. When the therapist does choose to share his or her feelings and thoughts with the patient, it is done with no ambiguity. The therapist is particularly sensitive to areas in which he or she disagrees with the patient. Although respectful of the patient's right to feel and think as an individual, the therapist can be clear with the patient about his or her own feelings and thoughts (avoiding the temptation to minimize disagreement by murky or evasive statements). As a therapist, one may choose to share personal material with a patient, but there is no therapeutic indication for lack of clarity.

Developing awareness of the process of facilitating autonomy is difficult. Often, a therapist needs to listen to tapes of interviews in order to discern the subtle ways autonomy may be either encouraged or discouraged.

AFFECT

Whether an interaction focuses on feelings or avoids them has profound significance. Most teachers of psychotherapy and researchers emphasize that learning that leads to change occurs most often in the context of affective arousal. The therapist needs to monitor the degree to which the expression and exploration of feelings are encouraged, the level of both cognitive and affective empathic responsiveness, and the degree of a personal sense of emotional guardedness. Perhaps one helpful indicator is whether or not there is at least one moment during each psychotherapy session when the therapist feels deeply moved and with the patient. This suggests that affective issues are very much a part of the interaction, for high levels of patient's expression of feeling without a significant affective response within the therapist tells us little about the process of the therapy.

These eight qualities of the interaction (cadence, depth, distance, focus, power, negotiation and task efficiency, autonomy, and affect) do not exhaust the ways in which the therapist may monitor the process of the therapeutic interaction. They do, however, represent a sufficient range of observations to insure a reasonably adequate awareness of the process. They pose considerable difficulty for the beginner. Observations about the patient may be easy; awareness of one's self and the use of this awareness in psychotherapy are more difficult; monitoring an intricate interaction in which one is a participant often seems like an overwhelmingly involved task. The eight qualities of the process are of different levels of complexity, and require great sensitivity. It is hoped that this introduction early in the psychotherapeutic careers of the students will provide an experience upon which subsequent learning and growth may occur.

REFERENCES

1. LUBORSKY, L., "Helping Alliances in Psychotherapy." In: J. L. Claghorn (ed.), *Successful Psychotherapy*. New York: Brunner/Mazel, 1976.
2. STRUPP, H. H., *Psychotherapy: Clinical, Research, and Theoretical Issues*. New York: Jason Aronson, Inc., 1973.
3. KNIGHT, E., "The Therapeutic Alliance." Paper presented at Timberlawn Psychiatric Hospital, Dallas, Texas, March, 1977.
4. LEWIS, J. M., BEAVERS, W. R., GOSSETT, J. T., and PHILLIPS, V. A., *No Single Thread: Psychological Health in Family Systems*. New York: Brunner/Mazel, 1976.
5. BEAVERS, W. R., *Psychotherapy and Growth: A Family Systems Perspective*. New York: Brunner/Mazel, 1977.
6. CHESSICK, R. D., *How Psychotherapy Heals*. New York: Science House, 1969.
7. CHESSICK, R. D., *Why Psychotherapists Fail*. New York: Science House, 1971.
8. CARKHUFF, R. R., *Helping and Human Relations*, Vol. I & II, New York: Holt, Rinehart & Winston, Inc., 1969.
9. KAGAN, N., *Studies in Human Interaction*, 3 Vols., U.S. Dept. H.E.W. (ED107946), December, 1967.
10. HENRY, W. E., SIMS, J. H., SPRAY, S. L., *The Fifth Profession*. San Francisco: Jossey-Bass, 1971.

CHAPTER 7

++

Interventions

++

++

The therapist has three sources of data in each psychotherapy session: the patient, the therapist, and the nature of their interaction. Much of the work of therapy involves a type of intense listening to these multiple sources of data. In my opinion, the ability to be involved with another in this way does not come naturally; it is an acquired skill that consumes considerable energy. During the course of a single session, a therapist will experience three distinctly different types of mental activity: intense listening, a more detached and analytic activity, and the less structured empathy. I believe that these three types of mental activity cannot go on concurrently, for they are different ways a therapist experiences himself or herself and another. He or she may move to or be pulled from one type of activity to another, often without any sense of conscious decision. On other occasions, the transition from one to another is the result of a conscious decision set in motion by questions that occur silently. "Where is he (the patient), what is he experiencing?" "What in the world does that mean?" "Why do I feel sad?" "Is there more distance today?"

Although each of the three forms of activity can be intense, there is a passive element to each. I use passive here because the activity is mental—not doing anything that intervenes in or impacts on the situation. This willingness of the therapist to accept this type of intense yet passive situation is difficult for a beginning therapist who struggles to varying degrees with the need to be active and feel masterful. For this reason, it is helpful early in the seminar to introduce several of the psychotherapeutic skills that acquaint the student with active intervention. Perhaps the easiest and most active skills to introduce early are confrontation and clarification. However, regardless of which intervention skills are introduced, it seems important for most students to experience this type of activity during the initial stages of learning.

There are many intervention techniques, and in this seminar for beginning therapists only a small number are introduced, with the assumption that the students' repertoire and expertise will increase in advanced seminars and individual supervision. Those which are introduced include: 1) facilitating deeper exploration; 2) focusing on the here-and-now of the therapeutic relationship; 3) confrontation; 4) clarification; and 5) interpretation.

FACILITATING DEEPER EXPLORATION

Much that the therapist does during the interview is meant to facilitate increasing self-exploration on the part of the patient. Responding empathically, for example, serves as a powerful stimulus to many patients. Reflective statements that may not, in themselves, communicate significant empathy can encourage patients to move on in their self-explorations. Interpretations may not only increase the patient's insight, but also promote further exploratory work. In addition, there are some relatively simple facilitators that the beginner needs to be acquainted with and begin to use. Simple requests to proceed such as "go on," or "tell me more" indicate to the patient that his or her feelings and thoughts are relevant, important, and of interest to the therapist.

They are not meant to select the focus, but request the patient to proceed wherever the patient's thoughts, feelings, and fantasies lead. At the same time, they do not necessarily "push" for greater depth.

The therapist's language is an important element in facilitating increasing depth of self-exploration. The seminar places heavy emphasis on the therapist's use of everyday language. Highly intellectualized or abstract language can be a potent deterrent to the patient's exploration. Its message may be interpreted as "let's keep our discussion civilized, erudite (and away from feelings or socially unsanctioned topics)." Carkhuff (1) has addressed this issue in his discussion of concreteness. At high levels of concreteness, the therapist demonstrates a willingness to meet the patient where he or she "is" and to interact with a language that is direct and closely related to the patient's actual experiences. This takes a degree of sensitivity and careful perception of the patient's style of expression. I do not suggest, however, that a therapist can "force" a level of language with which he or she is not comfortable. This may appear to be artificial and often is easily detected by, and confusing to, the patient. In the beginning, the therapist should be as concrete and specific with his or her language as possible while remaining genuine. If it is comfortable for the therapist, it is often helpful to use the patient's level of language. Highly intellectualized language should be avoided. Occasionally, a student appears to cling to a highly stylized, abstract, and intellectual form of speech. In my experience, such students are usually anxious and significantly obsessive. If they are unable to resolve the anxiety and obsessiveness as the result of participation in the seminar, I may advise individual psychotherapy or psychoanalysis if they wish to pursue careers which include doing intensive psychotherapy.

The most active intervention designed to increase the depth of patient self-exploration is the therapist's focusing a response on segments or parts of the patient's communications that appear (to the therapist) to have a high potentiality for deeper meaning. An example follows:

Patient: The whole family disapproved and were very bitter with me. It was a terrible time. My father said it was cheap. They just went on and on with their criticism.

Therapist: They all let you have it . . . Father, in particular, thought it was cheap . . .

Patient: . . . yeah . . . it hurt him maybe more than the others . . . he felt we had kind of a . . . special relationship.

This sample, focusing on an aspect of the patient's statement that the therapist felt had a high potential for exploration in the area of the patient's relationship with her father, led to subsequent discussion of a special and highly charged relationship. It is to be noted that the therapist did not introduce the topic, but phrased the response in a way that focused this exploration by responding to a particular aspect of the patient's statement. The beginning student is taught that, under most circumstances, it is more helpful to respond to an aspect of the patient's communication than it is to introduce a topic. If, then, the patient appears unwilling or unable to explore that aspect further, some degree of resistance may be inferred and should be noted by the therapist. It is considered well, however, to offer the patient several opportunities to move on with such an exploration. In observing interviews, the students are often surprised by the gentle persistence of many experienced therapists who know that one avoidance by the patient is not conclusive evidence of resistance.

An example of persistent, selective focusing follows:

Patient: My mother and sister would go out and leave me alone at night. I was scared and would get into bed and pull the covers up. Sometimes I would take food to bed and eat under the covers. (The patient is a depressed, obese woman.)

Therapist: You were left, and you were little and scared and under the covers would . . . eat.

Patient: Umhum . . . they went out a lot . . .

Therapist: It must have been scary . . .

Patient: Yeah . . .

Therapist: You felt alone . . .

Patient: Um . . . (tears) . . . I did, I did . . . I was only eight or nine . . . it was awful . . . . and . . . all I could do was pull up the covers and imagine I wasn't alone . . . and eat and eat.

This exploration and that which followed resulted from a gentle, persistent focusing by the therapist. There was a degree of patient resistance, but it was overcome without interpretation by the therapist's persistence in offering the patient continuous facilitation.

In this way, the students are introduced to the concept of resistance to exploration, and if there is evidence of a working alliance, they are encouraged to persist in their focusing before moving to interpreting the resistance. There are, however, several warning signals that should alert the therapist to the possibility that the repetitive focus is too frightening for the patient. One is a marked and unusual increase in patient resistance. Another is the sudden occurrence of clear disorganization in the patient's thought process. A third involves the intuitive nudge that the therapist gets that the exploration has moved too rapidly into areas that the patient is not ready for. This intuitive sense must be attended, although the therapist must have some idea that it is not he or she who is too anxious to proceed.

The seminar introduces this form of intervention, and the instructor takes notes of patient-therapist exchanges during the videotaped student interviews with the actor "patient" and during the interviews with actual patients behind the one-way screen. Critique of their use of this technique occurs, of course, during supervision of actual psychotherapy interviews. In the residency program in which this seminar occurs, the trainees' psychotherapy interviews are tape recorded routinely, which allows attention to this type of technical learning.

FOCUSING ON THE HERE-AND-NOW

Many psychotherapists suggest that one of the most important sources of learning occurs when the focus is on the here-and-now interaction of patient and therapist. Strupp (2), for example, in-

dicates that interpretations are more effective when they deal
with the immediate situation than when they concern the distant
past. The emphasis on "what is occurring now between us?" is a
direct example of the influence of the interpersonal school of psychotherapy. In my judgment, it has influenced other schools of
psychotherapy, and is one of the factors involved in the increased
general interest in the therapeutic alliance. Celani (3) has described hysteria, for example, from the interpersonal-communica-
tional viewpoint. Starting with the basic assumption of the interpersonal approach that all behaviors of individuals in interactions
represent attempts to produce in others an emotional state that
will elicit a predictable response, he suggests that the interpersonal message of the hysteric is, "I am a weak, helpless, frail child
and am at your mercy." This covert message produces an emotional climate in the listener that limits and directs the behavior
toward the hysteric. The responses of the listener confirm the
faulty self-perceptions of the hysteric. In this way, the hysteric
creates an interpersonal world that responds in a manner congruent with the feelings of weakness and powerlessness. Para-
doxically, such behavior, by structuring the relationship, is implicitly a powerful controlling device.

Coyne (4) has described depression in interpersonal terms. He
states that the depressive symptoms are attempts to elicit reassurance of the depressed person's worth and acceptability which,
however, become increasingly aversive to others who feel in-
hibited, irritated, and guilty. They continue to give verbal expressions of acceptance, but with a growing discrepancy between
the content and affective quality of their responses. This discrepancy validates the depressed patient's feeling that he is not
"really" accepted, and subsequently increases his communication
of lack of worth. As can be noted, this type of interpersonal behavior—like the hysteric's—is strongly controlling in the way it
patterns the relationship.

The works of Celani and Coyne are described here as examples
of the influence of this type of conceptualization of the interpersonal nature of psychopathological states. As this type of material has been understood more widely, there has been an in-

creasing emphasis on the need for psychotherapists to be sensitive to implications of the immediate psychotherapeutic interaction.

Kagan's research (5) also suggests that much of what is not talked about in psychotherapy concerns the here-and-now of the interaction. Pande (6), in what he describes as an Eastern interpretation of psychotherapy, suggests provocatively that Western emphasis on insight is a culturally appropriate and "magnificent ruse" for fostering a long-term, intimate relationship. There exists in Western culture "a need to find a shared task in order to offer intimacy and love." Pande goes on to state, "Both parties unwittingly set a task of nibbling away the iceberg of the 'unconscious,' but in a real sense they perhaps are only breaking the ice between themselves. The language is of understanding and insight, but the metalanguage is of love and human involvement" (p. 426).

Each of these trends suggests that beginning therapists should be encouraged to focus the psychotherapeutic exploration on the here-and-now. Carkhuff has termed this intervention "immediacy," and it represents the therapist's sensitivity to the patient's feelings about the therapist at the moment. For beginning therapists, it often represents a particularly anxiety-filled and difficult training experience. In part, this may represent the fact that it is very different from social intercourse. It seems, as a consequence, strange to be talking directly with another about what is going on right now between them. It also produces anxiety because the patient is, at such moments, not the traditional object of observation; rather the relationship itself is under scrutiny.

The students are taught that they should be sensitive to the possibility that much of the patient's behavior in therapy is both responsive to the real person of the therapist and potentially representative of a covert attempt to produce a predictable response. Patients may be more or less open in trying to talk about the relationship. At one level are situations in which the patient openly communicates feelings about the therapist. The students are introduced to this frequently anxious situation in the initial audio-taped patient stimuli statements, some of which are such direct confrontations. The tendency of most beginners is to avoid dealing with the interpersonal aspects and respond only in terms of the prevailing affect.

> *Patient*: We're not getting anywhere . . . you don't seem interested . . . it all feels hopeless to me.
>
> *Therapist*: You're feeling hopeless . . .

In this example, the beginning therapist responds by avoiding the overt interpersonal, here-and-now message. The students are taught that, although there may be valid exceptions, it is most often a mistake to respond in a way that avoids dealing with the affect in its here-and-now interpersonal context. In other words, the burden of responsibility is on the therapist to have a reason for evading the interpersonal aspect of the patient's statement.

There are less overt situations in which the patient may be talking directly about the here-and-now of the relationship. One such situation is when the patient is exploring his feelings about a class of persons to which the therapist belongs.

> *Patient*: I was angry at Doctor Jones. He didn't seem at all interested when I went in for my physical . . . doctors just don't seem to have much interest in their patients, and when it's me, I get angry . . .
>
> *Therapist*: Doctor Jones . . . doctors just aren't interested . . . I wonder, too, . . . are you feeling that here with me . . . a lack of interest?

In this example, the therapist was sensitive to the real possibility that the patient's feelings were connected to their relationship and responded in a way that offered that focus for exploration.

Another, and perhaps more subtle cue, is when the patient is discussing a certain feeling or general relationship pattern involving a number of other individuals.

> *Patient*: It just never seems to work out . . . it always ends up with my losing the relationship. My father left . . . every real friend I had somehow left me . . . and now Jack says he's going to Alaska.

> *Therapist*: It seems you feel left by everyone . . . I kind of
> have the nudge that maybe there's some of that going
> on now . . . are you feeling something of that here with
> me?

In this example, the therapist was responsive to the "always" in the patient's statement and, in very tentative terms, offered a focus on the here-and-now of the ongoing relationship.

The most encompassing assumption—which is the heart of the interpersonal technique—is that the central, underlying concern of all that the patient says is the here-and-now of the ongoing relationship. From this perspective, a therapist needs no suggestions, however subtle, that the patient may be trying to share something of the here-and-now—for the basis of therapy is the patient's attempt to structure the relationship in accord with his or her presumptions or distortions about the therapist. Although the seminar makes use of the interpersonal perspective, the position is extreme. Rather, the students are taught that one important frame of reference is what the patient communicates about the therapeutic relationship and, as a part of that, what the patient is trying to do "with" the relationship reflects more of the patient's past experiences than it does of the reality of the therapist. This, then, is transference—it is always present, active, and distorting. To bring it into focus and explore it—but not to encourage it—is central to the work of therapy. The therapist's sensitivity to and focusing on the here-and-now not only provides needed clarification of the patient's distortions, but may diminish the likelihood of a fully developed transference neurosis or psychosis.

This intervention, the active focusing on the here-and-now, requires the therapist to know a great deal about his own influence on the interaction in order that he or she can assess that portion of the patient's interpersonal reality accurately.

CONFRONTATION

Confrontation is one of the most active forms of intervention. It is defined differently by various writers, and Adler and Myerson (7) have clarified these differences in bringing together a collection of essays on the subject. Part of the difficulty is that the term is used to describe two very different forms of intervention—one of which can be called "routine confrontations," and the other "heroic" (8). In the seminar, it is suggested that the students consider the act of confronting as a continuum; at one end of the continuum are routine types of confrontation, and at the other end are heroic confrontations.

The continuum of confrontations from routine to heroic is influenced by the context—that is, the nature of the situation. In routine confrontations, the alliance is effective, and the therapist is attempting to deal with usual, everyday resistances to exploration. In heroic confrontations, the alliance is in trouble, and the therapist is attempting to deal with a massive and effective resistance to the entire treatment process. Routine confrontations are not meant to be shocking; heroic confrontations hope to. There is no threat implied in routine confrontations, whereas there is the implicit threat that the patient will lose the therapist at the core of a heroic confrontation. A heroic confrontation frequently involves considerable affective arousal on the part of the therapist; he or she is deeply concerned, frustrated, helpless, or angry. Routine confrontations rarely involve any significant degree of therapist's affective arousal.

Weisman (9) states that confrontation is a tactic of "undenial": Its purpose is to separate what a person is from what he seems to be or states that he is. As such, it is aimed at vulnerability and defensiveness. For this reason, psychoanalytic writers like Greenson (10) have considered routine confrontations as part of the analysis of resistance to be used by the therapist when he or she notes any evidence of protected vulnerability. Often, a sign of vulnerability is some discrepancy in the patient's communication. The discrepancy between the content and the affective components of a patient's exploration is, perhaps, the most common discrepancy and may call for a "routine" confrontation. Other discrepancies may involve obvious contradictions in the content of the patient's exploration, interruptions in the flow of the patient's speech, and differences in the patient's concept of himself and his behavior. In these and other discrepancies, there is an obvious resistance to exploration involving some degree of denial and vulnerability.

Heroic confrontations, on the other hand, occur rarely in the course of therapy. Corwin (8), who has reviewed the literature about this intervention, defines a heroic confrontation as "an emotionally charged, parametric, manipulative, technical tool demanded by the development of an actual or potential situation of impasse and designed ultimately to remobilize a workable therapeutic alliance." The purpose of such a confrontation is to make psychotherapy possible in a situation where the alliance has eroded away; in Corwin's terms, "the tide has turned against the analyst and his procedures." There is often an element of surprise, shock, or drama in the delivery of this type of confrontation and, implicitly or explicitly, the therapist suggests some action on his or her part. The confrontation arouses anxiety in the patient—often, the fear that the therapist will abandon him or her. The patient must do something or the relationship is to terminate. It is obvious that such interventions are used sparingly and only in situations that the therapist experiences as emergencies.

The residents are introduced to routine confrontations during the early portion of the seminar. The videotaped patient statements present several examples of obvious discrepancies between the content and affective components of the patient's communication. One young woman, for example, is discussing discrimination against women in the office where she works. She says that she is angry repeatedly, but throughout the entire videotape segment, there is a subtle smile on her face. Not all students perceive this discrepancy, and those who do frequently do not know how to deal with it. This becomes the initial opportunity to discuss routine confrontations.

An important aspect of teaching beginning therapists how to use routine confrontations is to suggest strongly that their manner is of critical significance. The students learn to confront in a manner that minimizes the likelihood that the patient will experience the confrontation as an attack. There must be an element of tenta-

tiveness to such confrontations—particularly if they occur during
the early stages of the alliance. ("I hear your concern about discrimination at the office and, although you say it angers you, I
think I see a faint smile.") In this way, the suspected underlying
vulnerability is brought out, but the therapist does not attempt
to impose his reality on the patient.

Heroic confrontations are introduced to the seminar group by
reviewing Corwin's work (8); there is no experiental exercise that
allows the student to practice or "get the feel" of this type of
intervention. I have been unable to find examples in the films of
other therapists, perhaps because such interviews are usually
"one-time" dialogues rather than interviews filmed during the
course of therapy.

It is anticipated that the students will continue to learn about
confrontation in discussing their tape-recorded psychotherapy
sessions with supervisors. The seminar, however, introduces this
form of intervention very early in their careers.

Examples of both forms of confrontation are presented. They
are taken from tape-recorded interviews.

Routine Confrontation

Patient: It was about the time my parents divorced . . .

Therapist: How did you feel about that?

Patient: What?

Therapist: What did you feel when your parents divorced?

Patient: Nothing . . . I felt nothing.

Therapist: Nothing . . . ?

Patient: No . . . I had no feelings . . .

Therapist: I think I see tears in your eyes . . .

Patient: Ah . . . no . . . well . . . perhaps . . . I did or do feel
    . . .

Therapist: It is painful . . .

Patient: (crying softly) I feel it now—like the world was
    ending and I was all alone . . .

In this example, the therapist confronted the patient with the discrepant messages—the verbal denial of feelings and the tears.

Heroic Confrontation

> *Patient*: . . . and then again last night I drank a fifth of scotch . . .
>
> *Therapist*: For several weeks it has been a fifth each night . . .
>
> *Patient*: Yeah . . .
>
> *Therapist*: We've talked about it . . . and yet you seem unable or unwilling to stop.
>
> *Patient*: It seems that way . . .
>
> *Therapist*: I'm beginning to feel we must do something about it . . .
>
> *Patient*: What do you mean?
>
> *Therapist*: Ah . . . we'd better . . . consider hospitalization.
>
> *Patient*: I won't go into a hospital.
>
> *Therapist*: Well—we must do something.
>
> *Patient*: No hospital . . .
>
> *Therapist*: Perhaps not—but—I'm beginning to wonder if we should continue our sessions . . .
>
> *Patient*: What do you mean?
>
> *Therapist*: I am beginning to feel that you must either stop drinking—or go into a hospital . . . or we should stop.
>
> *Patient*: You would do that?
>
> *Therapist*: Yes—it doesn't make any sense to continue like this . . .

In this interchange, the therapist confronted the patient with the impasse in treatment associated with the patient's drinking. The threat of abandonment was explicit.

CLARIFICATION

The term clarification is used in the seminar to describe the therapist's attempt to highlight certain patterns or trends in the patient's communication. It does not deal primarily with unconscious material and, as a consequence, does not ordinarily invoke specific resistances. If the clarification is relevant, it may, as Bibring (11) has pointed out, produce a sense of mastery—rather than danger—within the patient.

Although clarification may be brief, the students learn that their summarizing statements represent common opportunities for clarification. The patient, for example, may have finished a lengthy exploration and become silent. The student may wait, reflect the primary affect, comment on the resistance to further exploration, or offer a clarifying summary.

> *Patient*: After mother died, things were bad ... the economy was off, jobs were scarce ... gee ... we didn't know all the time if there would be enough to eat. Daddy was sick, but he tried ... He never was very strong ... and the plant where he worked was a terrible ... and ... well, after that ... he just left. The three of us were all alone and the welfare people arranged for a placement ... my brothers went together but I was sent to this family by myself ....
>
> *Therapist*: So ... first your lost Mother, then Daddy left ... and then you lost your brothers ...

In this example, the therapist does not introduce any new material or approach the repression of the underlying sadness and rage, but offers a summary that clarifies the major theme of the patient's exploration.

INTERPRETATION

Perhaps the intervention that provokes the most disagreement among the various schools of psychotherapy is interpretation. Its place at the center of psychoanalysis and psychoanalytic psychotherapy is well established. The existential school approaches something of the meaning of interpretation in its concept of "translation." The interpersonal school suggests that, rather than interpret, one must act against the patient's projections in the here-and-now of the ongoing relationship.

Bibring (11) indicates that interpretation refers to unconscious material, including mechanisms of defense, hidden meanings, and unconscious connections. By its very nature, interpretation goes beyond the data of the interview. I believe it is "going beyond" the data that may lead to confusion. If the interpretation is, indeed, a hypothesis about underlying meaning, defenses, or connections, it needs to be presented to the patient as a hypothesis. Stocking (12) has emphasized this point in distinguishing interpretations from confrontation: The former involves sharing a hypothesis that requires further validation, while the latter presents the patient with an already defined reality.

The seminar only introduces the role of interpretation to the students and relies on advanced seminars and individual supervision to develop their skills in interpretive work. We do not approach the complex issues of depth and timing of interpretations. Only two aspects of interpretation are dealt with in the seminar. First, the students are encouraged to frame their interpretations in tentative language and avoid any suggestion of mind reading or intrusiveness. A therapist cannot really know what is going on within the patient without exploration. For the therapist to suggest that he or she really *knows* is to communicate a level of power that is unattainable. In order, therefore, to avoid misrepresenting the power to know, it is wise to couch interpretive work in the language of hypotheses. This can be done by the use of introductory phrases like, "I've wondered if . . . ," "It seems that . . . ," "One possibiilty might be . . ." Although interpretive work is almost always more than a single statement, and actually occurs over extended periods, the use of tentative language throughout minimizes the risk of establishing the therapist as omnipotent. It is, however, precisely the opportunity to interpret that can seduce the beginning therapist to a display of power (often as respite from insecurity and uncertainty), and students occasionally make interpretive proclamations as if they held the chalice of Truth.

A second general principle of interpretive work that is emphasized in the seminar is the need to have the patient do as much of the interpretative work as possible. People in general, and patients in particular, value that which they have worked to obtain. Interpretive insight should, under optimal circumstances, be experienced by the patient as something he has accomplished rather than as something given by a powerful therapist. Therefore, the students are taught that the opening phases of an interpretive period are oriented around the therapist's asking, "How do you put that all together?" or "Can we understand the meaning of this—what are your ideas?" This emphasis not only shares the responsibility for the interpretive work, but is respectful of the patient's capacity to understand the meaning of his or her own behavior. If, however, the patient is unable to proceed, the students are encouraged to clarify the aspects of the patient's communication that led to the therapist's hypothesis and request the patient to proceed with the interpretive work. "Well, considering what we've noted about . . ., does something else come to mind?" If the patient cannot proceed, the therapist must then decide whether to deal with the remaining resistance or to offer the patient his or her (the therapist's) hypothesis.

This emphasis on joint or mutual interpretive work encourages the patient to experience therapy as a cooperative venture. Indeed, in all of the interventions introduced in the seminar, the emphasis is on working collaboratively. Because these interventions are at the heart of the therapist's expertise, they are often seen as part of his or her power. The therapist, while using very real expertise, wishes to minimize the power differential. Interventions are, therefore, a critical aspect of the establishment of a balance of power. If the therapist routinely focuses, confronts, clarifies, and interprets in a way that suggests he or she holds the key to reality or the truth, a relationship is established along an omnipotent-impotent axis. Only relatively slight growth can occur in the "impotent" one in such situations. If, however, the therapist is attentive to the difference between the role as expert and interpersonal power, he or she can use these interventions in ways that emphasize the patient's capabilities. In doing so, the therapist intervenes effectively and, at the same time, provides a context in which maximum change and growth can occur. It is this possibility that the seminar tries to impart to its students. The matter of full technical expertise with these interventions can come with subsequent experience and learning. What is hoped is that the student will develop both an initial familiarity with the specific interventions and an attitude about their use that is in keeping with the commitment to provide patients the maximum opportunity for growth.

REFERENCES

1. CARKHUFF, R. R., *Helping and Human Relations*, Vol. I & II. New York: Holt, Rinehart & Winston, Inc., 1969.
2. STRUPP, H. H., *Psychotherapy: Clinical, Research, and Theoretical Issues*. New York: Jason Aronson, Inc., 1973.
3. CELANI, D., "An Interpersonal Approach to Hysteria." *American Journal of Psychiatry*, 133:12, December, 1976, pp. 1414-1418.
4. COYNE, J. C., "Toward an Interactional Description of Depression." *Psychiatry*, 39:1, 28-40, February, 1976.
5. KAGAN, N., *Studies in Human Interaction*. 3 Vols., U.S. Dept. H.E.W., (Ed107946), December, 1967.
6. PANDE, S. K., "The Mystique of 'Western' Psychotherapy: An Eastern Interpretation." *Journal of Nervous and Mental Disease*, Vol. 146(6), June, 1968, pp. 425-432.
7. ADLER, G., and MYERSON, P. G. (eds.), *Confrontation in Psychotherapy*. New York: Science House, 1973.
8. CORWIN, H. A., "Therapeutic Confrontation from Routine to Heroic." In: G. Adler and P. G. Myerson (eds.), *Confrontation in Psychotherapy*. New York: Science House, 1973.
9. WEISMAN, A., "Confrontation, Countertransference, and Context." In: G. Adler, and P. G. Myerson (eds), *Confrontation in Psychotherapy*. New York: Science House, 1973.
10. GREENSON, R. R., *The Technique and Practice of Psychoanalysis*. New York: International Universities Press, 1967.
11. BIBRING, E., "Psychoanalysis and the Dynamics of Psychotherapy." *Journal of the American Psychoanal. Association*, 2:745-770, 1954.
12. STOCKING, M., "Confrontation in Psychotherapy: Considerations Arising from the Psychoanalytic Treatment of a Child." In: G. Adler and P. G. Myerson (eds.), *Confrontation in Psychotherapy*. New York: Science House, 1973.

CHAPTER 8

++

Overview and

Other Directions

++

++

The seminar described in these pages has evolved over a considerable number of years and continues to change in scope and detail. At the core, it addresses the issue of the balance of intimacy and detachment required to be an effective psychotherapist. It started with a central concern about the neglect of affect in psychotherapy and, as a consequence, during its early years the major focus was on empathy. This starting point has been balanced during more recent years by increased emphasis on the skills of detachment. The exercises designed to augment the student's capacities for the particular type of disciplined intimacy required by the role of psychotherapist have included empathy, warmth, respect, genuineness, and self-disclosure. The exercises aimed to increase the skills of detachment have included three groups: The first and more-or-less traditional observational skills include listening for associations, the recognition of major themes and

157

affects, the recognition of signs of arousal or conflict, the identification of mechanisms of defense, the increased sensitivity to
nonverbal communication, and the capacity to synthesize observations into a tentative hypothesis or clinical formulation. The second group of skills of detachment concerns the process of the
interaction itself and the capacity to monitor the process through
attention to several of its formal or structural properties (cadence, depth, and distance). The third group of skills of detachment involves psychotherapeutic interventions. The seminar con-
centrates on the facilitation of deeper exploration, focusing on
the here-and-now of the patient-therapist interaction, confrontation, clarification, and interpretation.

These discrete psychotherapeutic skills are of differing orders
of complexity. For most beginning therapists, those that are concerned with intimacy are the most difficult. However, when the
students understand the importance of skills related to intimacy
and have the opportunity to experiment with them within the
seminar, they become less frightening. The skills of detachment
are somewhat easier to learn. Here the patient is more the object
of the therapist's observations and interventions. This stance is
more familiar to the beginning therapists. Early, though, the students are introduced to the profound impact of the here-and-now
interaction on the patient's behavior. The need to learn to judge
one's impact and to avoid either inviting or prohibiting certain
patient behavior and then labeling it as characteristic of the
patient is a major task associated with the skills of detachment.

The therapist's variables or skills are derived from different
sources. Some originate in the objective-descriptive tradition or
school, whereas others come from psychoanalysis, interpersonal
psychiatry, existential psychiatry, or the research study of competent human systems. I think this borrowing is justified on at
least two grounds. The first is the current state of process research
in psychotherapy. We know that psychotherapy can be very potent, but do not know the ways in which it exerts its influence.
This inadequacy in current knowledge may be corrected by future
research, but until that day, it seems wise to introduce beginners
to as broad a spectrum of variables and skills as possible. This is

particularly appropriate if one organizes the skills around a balance of intimacy and detachment. Many writers from diverse schools of therapy agree that a flexible balance in these two very different ways of relating is necessary.

The second justification is that most experienced psychotherapists evolve their own personal amalgam of skills. The relative weights of different skills will vary from therapist to therapist. At this point in time, the theory and techniques of psychoanalytic psychiatry are dominant, but the past several decades have been marked by an increasing impact from both existential and interpersonal psychiatry. The impression that there are few purists suggests further justification for teaching a broad range of skills. It is hoped that with increasing experience, psychotherapists will come to use different skills or combinations of techniques with different patients, depending on the nature of the patient's psychopathology.

The seminar introduces the students to the complicated realm of the therapist's values and their influence on the way each perceives and responds to patients. The goals of this aspect of the seminar are to sensitize the students to the necessity of dealing with values openly and to extinguish whatever remnants there are of the romantic illusion that psychotherapy can be independent of the therapist's value orientations.

In its emphasis on the opportunity to use specific techniques, the seminar is committed to an experiential type of learning. Although there is considerable cognitive or didactic input, more than anything else the students are involved actively in doing, practicing, and correcting errors. The seminar, as a whole, is an experience that arouses the students' affect considerably. Although much of the affect is painful, it is the seminar's premise that learning is more apt to be valuable and retained if it occurs in such a context. What is sought in the seminar is the most effective balance of experiential and cognitive learning.

The seminar is seen as complementary to the other two primary ways of learning to be a therapist—individual supervision and personal psychotherapy or psychoanalysis. The seminar itself is concerned with the teaching and learning of psychotherapy skills that are frequently unattended in training programs. Indeed, it is my opinion that technique is the most neglected aspect of training psychotherapists.

The seminar shares commonalities with the approach of Ornstein and his colleagues (1), but there are major differences also. Those teachers agree that students' talents for observation, evocative listening, empathy, and introspection need broadening, deepening, and sharpening. Their approach is an integrated series of courses throughout the entire training period that are intended to free the students' native abilities. In their wish to avoid imitative learning, they emphasize the principles, logic, and theory behind a particular technique rather than the technique itself. In the effort to avoid the students' identification with the teacher, they minimize the teacher's role as a source of active encouragement and demonstration. The seminar, as described in this text, is concerned centrally with instruction and experience in technique, but includes also a significant emphasis on theory and principles. It is not, in my experience, an either/or situation. I have been less concerned with the danger of imitation because I believe there is something of that process in the very early stage of all learning. What would be of concern would be evidence that either the students' personal growth or evolution as therapists remained at an imitative level—that they failed to achieve the level of independent thinking that Ornstein and his colleagues articulate so clearly. It appears that the seminar described shares with Ornstein's teaching approach both agreement about the nature of the teaching problems (the development of students' native abilities) and the goals of learning (the achievement of the capacity for independent thinking). The processes used in the attempt to get from the problems to the goals are, however, very different.

IMPLICATIONS OF THE SEMINAR FOR OTHER HELPERS

The seminar has been described as it is taught to first-year residents in psychiatry and graduate students who function also as psychotherapists. I have experimented, however, with presenting shorter and appropriately modified seminars to other groups.

Variations of the seminar have been addressed to nonpsychiatric physicians, clergymen, nurses, medical students, and business executives. The duration of such seminars has been from 12 to 50 hours. Such seminars require a clear definition of the goals of each seminar. It has been my experience that the difference between training psychiatrists, psychologists, and social workers and training others who are involved with patients in ways that may have profound therapeutic impact involves the fact that the former group must have a knowledge of psychopathology. This includes psychodynamics, developmental aspects of the human life cycle, and a host of other factors. Members of the other helping groups may come to be professional therapists, but there is little about their disciplines' education that provides them with a comprehensive knowledge of psychopathology. This observation leads to basic changes in the seminar when it is offered to such groups. I have preferred to call this training "collaborative problem solving" rather than training in psychotherapy skills.

Collaborative problem solving teaches students to be of maximum help to others through interviewing techniques that facilitate the other individual's exploration of a problem. The exploration is observed to lead often either to a redefinition of the problem or to a much clearer understanding of the original problem. The students are taught to listen for affective messages from the person and to respond empathically whenever possible. The empathy taught to such students is primarily that defined in Chapter 2 as cognitive empathy. Students are encouraged to learn this skill because it is the hallmark of any helping relationship and is the most important way one person can encourage another to explore himself or herself. It has been helpful to use some of the same audio- and videotaped stimuli in these training seminars as used in the seminar for professional therapists. In other situations, however, other stimuli tapes have been created that are appropriate to the context in which the particular students work.

The initial portions of these seminars involve helping the students give up a sole reliance on a directive interviewing style. It is a source of personal amazement that, regardless of background and education, students come to such a seminar with identical interviewing approaches. They ask a series of focused questions that direct the flow of the interview. As they begin to experiment with a less directive style it becomes evident that the directive approach minimizes their own anxiety. Despite the observation that it is often possible to learn more about another and his or her problems by encouraging exploration in less directive ways, most students experience a strong pull to the directive style with its focused questions and answers. Even after achieving competence with collaborative interviewing (and, therefore, having two different interviewing approaches to use in different situations), students find themselves reverting to a directive style when they are uncertain, anxious, or afraid. The dangers of a sole reliance on the directive approach include the failure to define clearly the problem that brings the other to the helper's attention. This is because so often the other's initial presentation does not present the problem clearly. The directive approach, with so much reliance on the helper's thoughts in determining what is to be talked about, also may lead to self-fulfilling hypotheses and premature closure on the part of the helper.

The students are introduced to the concept that collaborative problem solving involves sharing both their power and the responsibility for outcome with the other. This involves a number of critical issues, including respect for the subjective views of the other and a commitment to negotiation as the primary basis for settling differences.

Students are encouraged to accept the results of their exploration with the other without any attempt to infer deeper meaning. There is no attempt to probe for underlying needs, conflict, or defenses. This is one of the major differences between the exploration of a professional therapist and that of other helpers. It is an attempt to help another define more clearly a conscious problem or problems with a helping other. It is when there is the sense that the "real" problem has been clarified that the collaborative problem process moves on to the phase of option-clarifying. In this stage, the helper encourages the other to explore and list solutions to the clarified problem. Only after a major effort has been made to elicit as many options as possible from the other does the helper add suggestions.

In collaborative problem solving, the stages of exploration and option-clarifying are taught with considerable structure, utilizing a variety of experiential exercises. Sensitivity to affective messages is emphasized through the use of taped stimuli, role playing, and demonstration by the instructor of both collaborative and directive interviewing styles. A particularly helpful exercise involves interrupted role playing. One participant is given a "problem," and another participant plays the role of helper without knowing the problem. As the role playing goes on, the instructor interrupts and "stops the action" from time to time. He then may ask the observers to critique the exploration or request that the participant with the problem share with the group his feelings about the progress of the exploration. The instructor also adds his or her observations. If the exploration is going badly, the participants may be asked to start again or, if it is going well, to pick up at the point of interruption.

The students are taught to be aware of the process of the interactions they establish with others who come to them with problems. The emphasis here is solely on the cadence of the interview rather than including depth and distance as in the training of professional therapists. The cadence of a collaborative exploration is more likely to involve brief statements by the helper followed by longer statements by the other.

The issue that is raised most frequently by the students is that the time required for collaborative exploration may not be available in their situations. Often, it does take longer, but has the advantage of offering the possibility of defining the problem more accurately. It also leads often to the other person's feeling that his or her feelings and ideas are respected. If he or she is involved actively in both the exploration and the option-clarifying, then whatever solutions emerge are his or her own as much as or more than the helper's. There is a greater possibility that the problem can be dealt with in one or a few sessions rather than becoming chronic and repetitious.

The seminar has been well received by primary care physicians and ministers. These are the two groups of professionals to whom many people turn when they face a personal crisis. A 20- to 30-minute interview format is suggested, and the participants report that it is a practical approach for them. In this regard, the seminar for these groups has some similarity to the work of Balint (2) who has suggested that patients take life problems to physicians, and patient and doctor negotiate a mutually agreed upon illness. There is an obvious base of collaboration in the doctor-patient relationship.

Nurses have responded enthusiastically to this training. For the most part, my experience has involved psychiatric nurses who, too often, are expected to be therapeutic in their relationships with clinic or hospital patients without being provided with a structure containing well-defined and appropriate skills. The seminar offers them both a framework and experiential exercises that lead to a sense of familiarity with specific techniques.

Recently, the seminar has been offered to executives of a single corporation on an experimental basis. A 32-hour format has been used, and we have been able to document the participants' increased communication skills as a result of the seminar. The participants, all of whom were chosen on the basis of their demonstrated corporate competence, were enthusiastic about the experience and its usefulness in their dealings with people with whom they worked.

In all these seminars, it is important to acquaint the participants with behavioral clues that suggest serious underlying problems that need to be referred to other appropriate helpers. It is also necessary to introduce them to the concept of resistance to exploration and, if resistance is strong and enduring, the impossibility of involving the other in meaningful exploration. There is also a need to teach students when collaborative exploration is contraindicated. This involves those infrequent situations when a person's level of functioning is so impaired as to constitute a real threat to his life or the lives of others. The need for the helper to intervene in a way that assumes nearly total responsibility for the other person—at least, for a brief period—is stressed in such situations. In a way somewhat comparable to work with patients, the executive deals sometimes with problems of such magnitude that he must define the problem as he sees it and move to effective action without emphasis on collaborative work with others. The distinction between those infrequent situations and those that are met best by a collaborative approach is, of course, the mark of the expert and mature helper. What is offered in these seminars is the concept that helpers from many disciplines can have several approaches, each of which has indications and contraindications for particular others.

THE CONTEXT OF THE TRAINING

It must be apparent that a training facility that makes the type of investment the seminar requires in terms of time, energy, and, ultimately, money must have a clear and strong commitment to the value of psychotherapy. The facility must be willing to make the substantial investment, not just in words, but in the practical realities mentioned above. First, it accepts the rather simple construct that beginning residents and graduate students are more student than they are providers of services. The two are not necessarily antagonistic, but (in my opinion) the balance should be weighted in the direction of learning. This means that time for seminars such as this one must be allotted and a smaller number of patients assigned to each student. It also means that the training facility must be willing to support this type of training, in part, before the student assumes the responsibilities of the role of the therapist with patients. This is difficult to accomplish in times when the valid needs of large groups of patients are emphasized. What must not be lost sight of, however, is the facility's responsibility to its patients. Providing patients with beginning therapists who have not had some introduction to both the *how* and *why* of psychotherapy is hardly fair to the patients. All this implies a clear commitment on the part of a facility to the patients' right to expect that their therapists—even if residents or graduate students—have a certain minimum level of psychotherapeutic competence.

There are two ways to teach swimming. One is to throw the students in the deep end of the pool and observe their wild attempts to reach the side. If they really seem about to drown, the instructor dives in and rescues them. The assumption is that out of the wild flailing about, valuable lessons will be learned and a sense of competence born. The other approach is to take the students into the shallow end of the pool, show them some swimming strokes, and let them practice in shallow water. When they have mastered basic skills, they can then move out into deeper water. In this approach, the instructor is in the water with the student and is involved actively in the students' learning. Now, both ways of learning to swim involve anxiety for the students— but, in my experience, the shallow-water approach presents less stress for them. Despite, then, the anxiety the seminar precipitates in the students, it represents an approach to training that allows for a beginning of the struggle for competence in the relative safety of a formal educational procedure. In this way, the seminar requires that the training facility hold as valuable the students' right to be treated with respect for their status as beginners.

The training facility must acknowledge and value openness in order both to allow and to nourish this type of seminar. The seminar itself involves a great commitment to practicing openly— that is, interviews are observed and often videotaped. Students and instructor respond to material with their own fantasies that are shared with the group. Errors are acknowledged and specific anxieties discussed. This type of educational process would have a difficult time flourishing in a training facility that did not encourage a comparable degree of openness. Openness can occur only in systems in which errors, mistakes, and failures are accepted as human frailties. The attempt, of course, is to keep blunders at the lowest level possible—but acceptance of their inevitability allows them to be shared with minimum loss of esteem.

The seminar also reflects something of the training facility's position on the state of current knowledge regarding effective psychotherapy. If there were not a shared belief that we have much to learn about the factors responsible for effective psychotherapy, there would not be the necessary tolerance and encouragement for such a seminar. This is because the seminar itself reaches out to all four major schools of psychiatry and the study of competent families as sources of valuable information. If there were within the facility a consensus that we really know what accounts for successful psychotherapy and the frequently associated commitment to one school or body of knowledge as "the only way," there would be little tolerance for a seminar that reaches as broadly as this one. In this manner, the facility must value research and have a willingness to distinguish what we know from what we think we know or would like to believe. Put another way, there can be little of a major reliance on an authoritarian belief system that prescribes rigidly a certain psychotherapeutic technique that is right for every patient.

These values—a real commitment to psychotherapy, the right of patients to anticipate a certain level of competence in their therapists, the right of students to have an opportunity to learn, a commitment to openness and the view that man is a mistake-maker, and an acceptance of the current state of our knowledge about effective psychotherapy—are factors within the larger context of the training facility that encourage the development of this type of seminar.

THE ROLE OF THE INSTRUCTOR

It is difficult for me to assess objectively the role that the instructor, both as a person and an expert, plays in the evolution of this type of seminar. Often, however, in presenting an overview of the seminar to faculty and staff in other training centers, I am asked a variety of questions about this issue. Perhaps the most common question involves how to deal with the intense affect regarding the instructor that the seminar precipitates. Let me, therefore, articulate my impressions of this complicated process. There is little doubt that the fact that the seminar is taught by the director of the residency training program itself intensifies the affective components of the participants' involvement. Whether this circumstance exerts a favorable or unfavorable influence on the quality of the participants' learning experience is difficult to ascertain. It has provided the instructor, however, with

the authority to construct the seminar and to assign the necessary curriculum time to it.

During the initial stages of the seminar, there is frequently
evidence of considerable uncritical acceptance of the instructor
and the content of the seminar. Later, for many of the participants, there is evidence of less involvement with pleasing the instructor and, for a few, considerable opposition to some of the
positions taken by the instructor. There may be increased tardiness and absences during this period. During later stages of the
seminar, there is evidence often of increased independent functioning by the students. Skynner (3) has summarized the developmental processes of groups and describes these three stages as
oral-dependent, anal-resistant, and genital-cooperative. During
the first stage, there is idealization of the leader and a wish to be
absorbed as part of his organization. The second stage of opposition and resistance to the leader is seen as a precursor of the independent, autonomous functioning that characterizes the third
stage.

This process is noted to one degree or another each year, but
it is surprising how different each group is. One year, for example,
the group moved rapidly through the first and second stages
and within several months appeared to be functioning with unusual autonomy. Another year involved a group that spent most
of the seminar time in a resistant phase characterized by an
undercurrent of opposition with more than usual tardiness and
absence. Within each group of students, there are individual differences in response to the instructor, but the group response
itself has been the more prominent force.

Perhaps the fact that there are a number of other faculty who
have close and prolonged contact with each resident dilutes somewhat the intensity of the individual emotional involvement with
the instructor. During the period of the seminar, for example,
each resident is assigned to a hospital unit and has a senior psychiatrist as a clinical supervisor. They make rounds, hold unit
meetings, meet families, and conduct team meetings together.
The individual resident may spend three to four hours each
day with the clinical supervisor, and often develops an intensely

cathected relationship with him. Rotation to another unit is experienced frequently as a significant loss by the resident.

At a conscious and deliberate level, I have tried to build my participation as instructor on the concept that how I behaved and what I did was as important as what was actually said. As a consequence, I strived for considerable openness regarding my mistakes and anxieties during interviews as well as sharing information about the kinds of affects and conflicts in patients that gave me greater than usual difficulty.

The seminar often requires a meticulous dissection of students' responses to stimuli or videotaped interviews, and it is important for the instructor to establish a model of close observation. This type of criticism of the beginners' efforts must be coupled with sensitivity to the students' anxieties as they approach the difficult task of learning to be therapists in a setting that involves making mistakes in front of others. It has occurred to me that the teacher of this type of seminar must communicate something of the same skills in teaching as are introduced to the students in their learning of psychotherapy. There is need for both the skills of detachment—observation and critical analysis—and the obviously human concern for the feelings of another as reflected by empathy, respect, and self-disclosure. In this suggestion I am, of course, noting what Marmor (4) has stressed for years: Psychotherapy, at its core, is a learning experience. It should not, therefore, surprise us to find similar processes in teaching and therapy.

OUTCOME OF THE SEMINAR

In restrospect, I wish that the seminar had been established on the basis of a research project. That thought remains a fantasy as the difficulties of finding control groups, defining and measuring outcome, and obtaining funding seem insurmountable. At this point, therefore, there are no data that demonstrate clearly that the seminar plays a role in the development of effective psychotherapists. The dilemma posed by lack of measurement of all educational processes has not been eased by this seminar. We continue to be burdened by our short-sightedness, to say nothing of the difficulties of encouraging funding agencies to support such studies. There are, of course, numerous research investigations regarding the outcome of psychotherapy (5), but none that I am aware of regarding the outcome of the training of psychotherapists.

As a consequence, there are available only the very impressionistic data from the participants—none of whom have learned from jumping or being pushed into the deep end of the pool and, as a consequence, have little of a contrasting experience. It is, perhaps, even reasonable to assume that having survived the seminar, they look back on it with the satisfaction of the military recruits who have survived basic training. It's not what they learned, but the surviving in itself that may be the fantasy behind the statements of former participants.

There are several aspects of the seminar that can be noted. Early attempts to measure empathy before and after this initial year of training show no evidence that it declines, as one study (6) of the impact of residency training suggested. Secondly, young professionals are introduced early in their careers to the value of openness about their work. My generation of therapists has not, as a group, been particularly enthusiastic about recording and sharing psychotherapeutic efforts with colleagues. Thirdly, the process of participating in such an open group has a generally cohesive impact on each class of residents. They seem better able to relate with less defensiveness to each other than other trainees whom I have come to know.

In presenting an overview of the seminar to the faculties of other training programs, I have been encouraged by those who have shared a sense of envy. "Why didn't I have the opportunity for that experience as a beginning resident?" has been remarked by several senior and respected teachers. This valuable input from others has been a source of encouragement in the evolution of the seminar.

The seminar continues to evolve and, it is hoped, will continue to change as new research data and teaching techniques tell us more about how to assist our students in their search for psychotherapeutic competence. Until, however, we know with greater certainty the most effective approaches to this task, we must continue to innovate and not accept too readily the ways of learning that we experienced as students. Many of us have had to struggle too hard and too long in our search for competence. Although there will always be some pain involved, we must remember that when anxiety exceeds a certain level, learning is diminished. To be a therapist is a noble aspiration, and that fire should not die in our students because we fail to protect it at its beginning from the winds of uncertainty, doubt, and fear.

REFERENCES

1. ORNSTEIN, P. H., ORNSTEIN, A., and LINDY, J. D., "On the Process of Becoming a Psychotherapist: An Outline of a Core-Curriculum for the Teaching and Learning of Psychoanalytic Psychotherapy." *Comprehensive Psychiatry*, Vol. 17(1), January/February, 1976, 177-190.
2. BALINT, M., *The Doctor, His Patient, and the Illness*. London: Pitman Medical, 1964.
3. SKYNNER, A. C. R., *Systems of Marital and Family Psychotherapy*. New York: Brunner/Mazel, 1976.
4. MARMOR, J., *Psychiatry in Transition*. New York: Brunner/Mazel, 1974.
5. MELTZOFF, J. and KORNREICH, M., *Research in Psychotherapy*. New York: Atherton Press, Inc., 1970.
6. KHAJAVI, F., and HEKMAT, H., "A Comparative Study of Empathy: The Effects of Psychiatric Training." *Archives of General Psychiatry*, Vol. 25, 490-493, 1971.

APPENDIX

+++

I. Training Exercises

A. Early Exercises

The initial experience focuses on Carkhuff's (1) 16 patient stimuli statements. These statements are recorded on audiotape and played to the group. After each of the recorded statements, the participants write what they would say in an attempt to be helpful to another person during an initial or early contact. Following the entire series of 16 statements, each of the participants reads aloud to the group his or her response. The instructor introduces the group to the concept of cognitive empathy during the discussion of the participant's responses. The emphasis is on how frequently the affective component of the patient stimulus was overlooked in the response.

The second series of ten tapes was created by the author and involves patient statements of greater difficulty. Each student responds to the series of tapes privately and orally. Responses are tape recorded and then spliced together so that all students' responses to the first stimulus can be listened to consecutively. The major focus of this exercise remains on cognitive empathy, but the constructs of warmth, respect, and genuineness are introduced through attention to the students' voice mannerisms.

The third exercise uses eight videotaped patient stimuli created by the author. These stimuli are responded to orally, and the responses are audiotaped. The taped responses are played and discussed by the group. In addition to cognitive empathy, warmth, respect, and genuineness, the responses offer the opportunity to introduce the group to observation of nonverbal clues, confrontation regarding discrepant messages, and the complex issue of therapist self-disclosure.

At this point in the seminar, the group views interviews of a patient by two psychiatrists. One interview is directive in the sense that the psychiatrist asks a series of specific questions regarding the patient's symptoms, family relationships, and childhood history. The second psychiatrist uses collaborative exploration and encourages the patient, in a less directive way, to explore areas of apparent affect. The instructor points out the advantages and disadvantages of each interviewing style and the videotapes are stopped frequently in order to raise questions about the process of each interview. The group is encouraged to note the examples of cognitive empathy, respect, warmth, genuineness, confrontation, nonverbal clues, and the use of therapist's self-disclosure. A particular focus, however, involves demonstrating that the collaborative exploration can be sustained throughout the interview, because until this time the students' experience with these techniques has been with brief segments of dialogue.

Two films are shown to demonstrate the difference in technique of two schools of psychiatry: psychoanalytic psychotherapy and Carl Rogers' existential type psychotherapy. The psychoanalyst maintains a cognitive and childhood-oriented perspective and interviews with frequent interpretations. Rogers' focus on feelings and his attempt to translate these feelings into words stands in sharp contrast to the psychoanalytic method. These films lead to a discussion of the four major schools of psychiatry and present the students with an early orientation regarding significant differences between the schools.

B. Practice Interviewing

The students practice the interviewing techniques they are learning by role playing. This is done in front of the group, and one student plays the "patient" and is given a "problem" that is unknown to the "therapist." The ten-minute role playing exercises center about the exploration of the assigned problem, and the group members and instructor are free to stop the role playing dialogue and question the participants. At a later stage in some groups, the students role play therapist and patient without an assigned problem to explore. Occasionally, this leads to the exploration of negative feelings about the seminar, exposure of mistakes, and threats to self-esteem.

Following this exercise, each student interviews the same actor "patient," and the interviews are videotaped. The actor or actress is instructed only that he or she has recently lost a lover, feels sad, and is having difficulty sleeping and eating. In all other ways, the "patient" is asked to be himself or herself and to allow each interview to evolve in whatever way seems natural. This exercise is one that arouses great anxiety in the students and, for some, this leads them to adopt a very formal and stereotypical, professional role and a directive, question-and-answer interviewing style. Others accomplish more skillful explorations. The videotaped interviews are reviewed by the group, and a number of teaching foci are apparent. These include a review of each student's developing interviewing skills, the impact of the interviewer's anxiety on the interview itself, the frequently interactional basis of the nonverbal communication (deleting the sound emphasizes how often the "patient" and the student move in what appear to be either complementary or parallel ways), and the strikingly different relationships and interactions established by different students.

Two new directions to the seminar evolve from the review of the videotaped interviews. One concerns the students' need to develop an awareness of the process of interactions. In subsequent sessions, they are introduced to cadence, depth, and distance as three formal characteristics of interactional process, and in subsequent interviews begin to observe these characteristics. Additionally, they are introduced to the system characteristics of competent families (2) that may be useful in evaluating psychotherapeutic processes.

The second direction growing out of the videotaped interview exercise and review involves mechanisms of defense and resistance. The actor or actress inevitably demonstrates resistance to certain explorations. The students have received no instruction at this point in the seminar on either the identification of mechanisms of defense or dealing with resistances. As a consequence, the interviewer gropes about during resistant segments of the interviews and expresses an interest in learning what to do. This leads the seminar to Vaillant's (3) work on mechanisms of defense and to an introduction to dealing with resistance.

C. Advanced Exercises

The earlier exercises have sensitized the participants to their impact upon the interaction. Two other exercises seem useful in this regard. The first is a Forced Fantasy Exercise in which the students respond to projected pictures by writing a fantasy that relates to the picture. The pictures are of various stages of human development and incorporate major life themes such as dependency, sexuality, aggression, and grief. As indicated in the text, this exercise often reveals something of the student's tendency to perceive certain themes idiosyncratically. The teaching message is that one's perceptions are a potent factor in precipitating certain interactional patterns, and each individual must come to know his or her tendency to perceive certain themes or images idiosyncratically. The instructor participates equally in this exercise and, in this way, encourages both openness and the concept that each individual is able to "see" and respond to some themes better than others.

Kagan's Interpersonal Process Recall technique is demonstrated as described in this text. This exercise leads to increased appreciation of the subtle changes in interpersonal distance that occur during an interview. The technique is time-consuming, and during some seminars I use the Interpersonal Process Recall tape from a previous seminar. The pace of the seminar varies from year to year. If a particular group of students is learning at a slower-than-usual rate, I delay the start of interviewing actual patients behind the one-way screen. Under usual circumstances, however, the seminar has proceeded to this interviewing phase before the students are assigned patients for formal psycho-therapy.

II. Interviews with Patients

The interviews are with hospitalized patients who know the interviews are observed and that their participation is part of a training procedure. Their consent to participate is voluntary and, on rare occasions, a patient will be unwilling. The student conducting the interview is asked to do an exploratory interview, and the patient is not known to the student prior to the interview.

The other students and the instructor sit behind the one-way screen and observe the 30-minute interview. Each student accepts the responsibility for monitoring one or more aspects of the interview. During the late stages of the seminar, a different student monitors all of the dimensions of the interview in an effort to teach students the skill of making numerous observations about discrete variables.

In addition to the emphasis on the skills concerned more with intimacy, there is a major focus on the development of the skills of detachment. These include the observations skills and the intervention techniques.. Observing students are encouraged to take notes and to document their observations as a base for any inferences about the patient.

The group is introduced to the process of making a clinical formulation and contrasts this formulation with that of the clinician treating the patient.

Each student does three to five interviews in rotation. The group offers support as well as confrontation. There is evidence of improved interviewing skills as a result of the confrontation by peers.

REFERENCES

1. CARKHUFF, R. R., *Helping and Human Relations*, Vol. I. New York: Holt, Rinehart & Winston, Inc., 1969, 115-123.
2. LEWIS, J. M., BEAVERS, W. R., GOSSETT, J. T., and PHILLIPS, V. A., *No Single Thread: Psychological Health in Family Systems*. New York: Brunner/Mazel, 1976.
3. VAILLANT, G. E., "Theoretical Hierarchy of Adaptive Ego Mechanisms." *Archives of General Psychiatry*, Vol. 24, February, 1971, 107-118.

INDEX

179